INTERMITTENT FASTING FOR SENIORS

THE COMPLETE GUIDE TO INTERMITTENT FASTING TO LOSE WEIGHT, FEEL MORE ENERGIZED, AND LIVE HEALTHIER LIVES AFTER 50

ANDREW JOHNSON

INTRODUCTION

Fasting is a staple of our ancestral history. Denying ourselves sustenance, especially in times of prayer, mourning, or as a form of sacrifice has been a tradition among many religions for centuries. Some religions even continue this practice annually.

Yet, outside of religious convictions, most people adhere to the belief that eating three meals a day is best for your metabolism. Eating breakfast, lunch, and dinner, at respectable times of seven, twelve, and six is the best way to stay healthy.

Enter **Intermittent Fasting.**

Intermittent Fasting is a growing trend that defies all of the timely conventions of a healthy eating cycle. This type of eating regimen does not dictate

what you should eat. Rather, Intermittent Fasting tells the participant **when** they should eat.

Instead of counting carbs, taking supplements, and buying overpriced dishes that taste more like the ghost of your favorite meal than the real thing, you get to eat food. Real food. Every day (if that is what you choose to do).

This is a guide to intermittent fasting and the incredible benefits it offers, specifically as it relates to seniors.

WHAT IS INTERMITTENT FASTING, AND WHY SHOULD YOU BE ON IT?

*I*ntermittent Fasting is defined by Michigan Medicine dietitian Sue Ryskamp as, "Individuals using specific periods of eating — typically within an eight-to-10 hour window — to lose weight."

THE BASIC THEORY behind Intermittent Fasting is simple and the cornerstone behind even marginally successful diets: Lessening a person's daily caloric intake will result in them losing weight and becoming healthier overall. This is especially true when the body is deprived of new calories for an extended period of time.

INTERMITTENT FASTING and Calories

. . .

A *CALORIE* IS a unit of measurement that relates to energy. The number of calories a food contains correlates to the amount of energy your body can receive from that food. However, the issue (weight loss and overall unhealthiness) comes from people taking in more energy than they can burn in a day. When a person is not burning that energy, it is stored and it is turning to fat. That is why many diets give participants a certain amount of consumable calories per day. If the dieter sticks to this they are giving their bodies fewer calories to work with, throughout the day. Eventually, this causes the body to pull from the reserve of energy that is stored as fat.

WHEN YOU FAST, your body is forced to use the energy you have already stored. This helps you lose weight, among other benefits.

INTERMITTENT FASTING WORKS SIMILARLY, except it forces your body to use that stored energy for a longer span of time.

WHEN PEOPLE REDUCE their calorie intake, each meal

will only provide them with so much energy. Our bodies are used to having an abundance of calories, which is why we gain weight. When those calories are lessened, the body takes from stored energy to make up the difference. Although, when a person is just lessening calories, the body only has to take from the reserve for a limited amount of time. If you are having three meals per day, the amount of food you are taking in is still interrupting the process of your body pulling from the reserves.

INTERMITTENT FASTING ELONGATES the timespan that the body has to collect energy from your reserves. Instead of starting and stopping multiple times per day, your body is either pulling energy from the reserves, or it is not. There is only one time per day (or per select amount of hours) that the body is changing its process. Thus, it is able to be more effective at both methods of collecting energy.

A STUDY CONDUCTED between 2011 and 2015 at the University of Illinois found that fasting was slightly more effective than regular caloric decrease. This is significant because while the difference was less than a percent, there were issues with the fasting group of the clinical trial that hurt the outcome. Throughout this trial, there was an excess of people dropping out of the trial from the fasting side. Adversely, the people who were simply decreasing their caloric intake remained in the study in much greater numbers. Yet, the average of this study was maintained and still surpassed the percentage of weight loss found in those that fasted, versus those who ate a low-calorie diet.

Fasting: Fact and Fiction

Fasting sounds far worse than it really is. The issue is much less about the diet itself and more about the stamina of the person who is dieting. Food is everywhere. Most of our socialization and most of the occasions that people look forward to having a centerpiece of food. Holidays, birthday parties, family get-togethers, even bars, usually have some kind of food. Plus, the portion sizes, especially in the United States, are astronomical. Everyone wants you to eat, drink, spend money, and be merry. Everywhere you turn, regardless of your age or where you live in the united states, is controlled by food.

THIS SOCIAL PRESSURE, in addition to the pressure of your own formed habits, makes dieting, never mind fasting extremely difficult. Fasting is an active, conscious decision. You are fighting everyone, including yourself when you decide to fast. It does not matter what age you are, we have trained our bodies to ask for far more than we need.

· · ·

BEFORE GETTING TOO deep into Intermittent Fasting, it is important to understand the truths behind the common myths surrounding fasting.

FASTING PUTS your body in starvation mode.

STARVATION IS NEVER healthy and should NEVER be considered, regardless of your age or level of fitness. Fasting is not starvation.

NEVERTHELESS, many people hear that people are fasting and it calls to mind the image of emaciation and the feeling of constant, terrible hunger. However, fasting is not meant to be punishment. Your body does not automatically default to starvation mode. Specifically, your body does not react to fasting by shutting down your immune system.

STUDIES HAVE CONCLUDED that people can actually fast between twenty-four to forty-eight hours and their metabolism will likely improve between 3.6 and 14 percent. The reason for this increase is that the body will begin to release higher levels of norepinephrine.

. . .

AGAIN, this is not starvation. Fasting is meant to train your body, to control your body, so that you regain control over your urges of consumption.

INTERMITTENT FASTING CAUSES your body to lose muscle mass.

INTERMITTENT FASTING DOES NOT MAKE your body lose muscle-mass. In fact, if the goal of your dieting is to gain muscle, as it might be for seniors, Intermittent fasting is a great way to do it. Many people report that through Intermittent Fasting, they are able to eat and even exercise less while gaining the same benefits.

THE SPAN of time your body needs to go without eating to start drawing from your stored energy is between eight and twelve hours. That is why going up to two days without eating is acceptable. Your body adjusts so that there is no permanent damage done to your body. Remember, your body needs far less than your body receives on a daily basis. We, as a society are gluttons. Older generations, with the exception of the extremely wealthy, as in some societies, obesity was a status symbol, ate far less than we do.

. . .

BREAKFAST IS **the most important meal of the day.**

BREAKFAST IS GREAT. There are a plethora of delicious options, which come with some of the best sides ever to dawn a plate. And, of course, this is the meal where coffee is the preferred beverage for most people.

YET, there is deception in our generalized idea of this "important" meal. This is another area where most people grew up believing an array of lies.

- **First:** Breakfast is not the most important meal of the day: Truth be told, breakfast is more or less, a useless meal, filled with calories that your body does not need. When we sleep, our body is in a fasting state. Therefore, if you drink a glass of water when you get up, (But, that doesn't mean we cannot enjoy these tasty breakfast calories at other times throughout the day.)
- **Second:** Skipping breakfast will not make you fat. This myth was started a few years

ago and, despite evidence to the contrary, it stuck with the majority of the public. The evidence that supports this myth was always due to a relativity than causality. Scientists found that when a person has breakfast, they normally stick to a daily routine. A routine is all around better for your body because it knows what to expect. Your body likes having a sense of what is coming next. However, that does not mean specifically that breakfast is a key element to this. After all, when a person commits to a schedule of intermittent fasting, they are adhering to a strict schedule too. (However, this one, research shows, does help you lose weight specifically when paired against breakfast-eating counterparts.) Essentially, though, you are still skipping a meal. Therefore, you are eating fewer calories than if you were to partake in a third meal.

- **Third:** Breakfast does not "kickstart" your metabolism. This is not how calorie consumption or burning work. Studies show that the number of calories burned within a twenty-four hour period is not affected by the time of day the calories are consumed. Intermittent fasting is in direct competition with this myth, as it is true that your body is in a state of fasting while you sleep. Eating obviously interrupts this state and therefore, breaks your fast.

YOUR BRAIN NEEDS a consistent supply of glucose to continue functioning:

THERE IS a belief out there that if you do not continue to supply your body with carbs, your brain will stop working. While, if you are hungry, it might feel as though your brain is refusing to work, it is perfectly fine. Again, your brain is trained to have a certain level of carbs per day. Almost like a spoiled child, if your body is used to a certain level of carbs and you are no longer supplying that level, your body reacts. (It is not hurt. It is not truly in need. Rather, it is having a temper-tantrum. Basically, it will get over it. This is simply a test to your endurance.

NOW, do you think you are expected to "get over it" by testing your pain endurance? No. Instead, drink a glass of water. The more likely culprit of your hunger pains is thirst. (Funny enough.) Thirst and hunger, according to studies, can feel a lot alike.

Weird, right? Well, instead of breaking your fasting cycle, try to drink a large glass of water. After you have finished the water, wait fifteen minutes. There is a good chance you will no longer feel the effects of being "hungry" because you were, indeed, thirsty.

HERE IS a list of symptoms that we are trained to believe is hunger but is really due to being thirsty:

- That gnawing, empty feeling in your stomach
- Stomach gurgling or rumbling
- Dizziness, faintness or light-headedness
- Headaches
- Irritability
- Lack of concentration
- Nausea
- Dry skin
- Feeling sluggish
- Dry-eyes
- Increased heart rate

AGAIN, we are trained to believe almost everything we feel is a result of a lack of sustenance. The reason, more likely than not, is that food is enjoyable.

Drinking water, which is actually far more impor-tant for your body, is not as exciting. There are so many different flavors of food. Water, while there are options, from putting lemon in your water to drinking club soda, is just not as satisfying.

THE TRUTH IS, the human body can live twice as long without food, as it can without water, as per the available information we have access to. It is much harder to pinpoint a timeframe for people now because it is unethical to starve people, (obviously). Therefore, the only information we have is the experiments that were done before ethics played a major role in scientific discovery and what scientists have observed from hunger strikes. From this infor-mation, scientists believe that without any suste-nance, whatsoever, the human body will survive eight to twenty-one days. With a consistent supply of water, though, the body will survive up to two months without food.

OF COURSE, there are many different factors that play into the specific person being able to live for a specific length of time.

HOWEVER, the point of this information is to explain

that hydration, although much less interesting than the consumption of food is far more important for survival.

Your body does not break down while fasting, it ramps up.

When people think of fasting, they immediately think of starvation. Starvation leads us to think about our bodies as meek and frail, unable to focus and barely able to function. In short, many people think that the body breaks down if it is subjected to fasting. However, that is not the case. If our bodies broke down in the days of the caveman, we would be extinct.

INSTEAD, our bodies ramps itself up when we do not have food. When we are fasting, our body builds up our basal metabolism and our levels of noradrenaline increase. This makes us feel energized and alert. This is likely why so many people report feeling energized in the middle of their fast.

External Factors that Contribute to Overeating

Eating can be a true form of torment for those that struggle with weight loss. People who try to eat healthily and eat less are constantly bombarded, both internally and externally by the idea that food is good. Friends, family, ads, social media feeds, our kitchens, and our own bodies remind us of the need for food, constantly. It is a struggle that is dealt with from the moment a person wakes up until they go to bed. The only relief is found when people go to bed; if they are not dreaming of food, that is.

In fact, personally, it never seems to fail; whenever I am trying to fast, or I am on a diet of any kind, there is always free food surrounding me. Not only is there the normal food temptations, but to make it even worse, it seems that everyone decides to *give* it away. Free samples abound and of course, it is everything that I love.

For most, this is an unfortunate cycle that haunts them every hour of their existence. Here are some of the most common external factors that contribute to overeating:

Social Media: Social media is filled with ads, food pics, restaurant reviews, and information about the different options for consumption. This initiates our "Visual Hunger" which goes into effect, regardless of whether we are actually hungry or not. All of these pictures look good and the reason is likely that they are almost all high-fat foods. According to Science Direct, high-fat foods are much more likely to trip a person's visual hunger sensors than low-fat foods.

(Which is kind of a given. There are not many people who would take an enticing picture of kale, much less many more viewers who would have a food orgy over it. Now, show that same person a triple-chocolate meltdown, with all the fixings, and...well, you get the picture.)

Regardless, the number of posts related to food is staggering and even if we are not hungry, we are constantly reminded of the presence and accessibility of food.

CONVERSATION: Even talking about food elicits a reaction of hunger. Reminding yourself of anything makes you more aware of its presence, (or the lack of it). Since food is generally a safe topic, many people discuss where they last had a good meal and what their favorite food is. When a person is in a social situation, where they might not know what to say, food is a great conversation starter. First of all, it's usually there and secondly, even if your opinion differs, with regard to the food, a passionate, yet friendly conversation can still take place.

SURROUNDINGS AND COMPANY: Everyone has got to eat. However, what you eat, who you eat it with, and how often you eat it is all related. Here is a quick experiment:

. . .

IF YOU GO out with friends, what comes to mind?

Most of us would conjure up our favorite dive, where we have spent many hours eating, drinking, and laughing.

IF YOU ARE ATTENDING A GALA, what comes to mind?

A gala is usually a formal occasion, so it is accompanied by a date, generally and you both are wearing your best. For the food, you might imagine a widespread of fancy finger food, possibly some of the fancier stuff like caviar, and possibly those little mini hotdogs.

IF YOU ARE GOING to a birthday party, what comes to mind?

Usually, for a birthday party, regardless of the age of the celebrator, the resounding constant for an American birthday party is CAKE! When you go to a birthday party, a wedding, or anything that is the least bit celebratory, a cake likely a cornerstone item of expected consumption.

ULTIMATELY, this is how our brains work. We have trained our brains and society has trained us to associate having a good time with food. That is not necessarily a bad thing, as food is the one language that everyone understands. Every human gets hungry and every human appreciates good food. The term "Breaking bread" with someone is traditionally a sign of friendship, comradery, and trust. Even the Bible offers a positive image of food...and all they reportedly had was carbs.

THEREFORE, it is not a wrong reaction, to want to include food in everything we do. However, the food that we have and the amount of food we consume is directly related to the people and places that surround us. If you are at The First Supper, you load up on carbs (and probably fish), if you go to a Vegan restaurant with a date (that you really like) you try to eat less and pick something healthy.

IF YOU'RE at a birthday party, you eat cake (and probably pizza). That is just the habit formed by generations of conventions.

LONELINESS: Yes, it is true that people tend to eat more when they are with people but being alone is also a possible trigger for overeating. When we are alone, we can convince ourselves of many different things. When we are alone, we are our true selves. Being lonely will make people feel even worse, thus intensifying feelings that turn to overeating.

SOMETIMES, it is boredom that causes us to eat. While this is not a particularly terrible emotion, it can lead to consuming far more than we need. Boredom can convince us that we need something to do. Thus, we talk ourselves into being hungry. This reward of food trains our body to look toward food as an escape from boredom. This quickly becomes a habit and therefore, at the first sign of boredom, your body will tell you it is "hungry" so that you have an easy escape from the discomfort of having nothing to do.

WHEN WE ARE LONELY, however, that feeling of boredom quickly turns to depression. This is a serious issue that many people try to mitigate by eating. Some people feel like they are filling a void with food and some people find it comforting. Either way, it is doing nothing positive for your body.

THE PATH OF LEAST RESISTANCE: Humans are hard-wired to pick the path of least resistance. Of course, this is not a trait that is exclusive to humanity. Yet, due to our being more complex than other species, this causes more issues for us than other animals. According to an article in Psychology Today humanity is wired to convince ourselves that the easiest way to achieve a goal is the best way. The reason is that it takes less energy. Psychology calls this type of thinking a branch of "Cognitive Dissonance". However, the more common term for this is laziness. Unfortunately, even our own mind tricks us into thinking that the more difficult task must be wrong because it is not easy. In times like these, our mind makes it incredibly easy to focus on all the ways the path of least resistance is the right call; even if we know it is not.

IRONICALLY, if the constant dangling of food was not torturous enough, people who struggle with weight and those who are trying to be healthy are also plagued with the reminder to eat well. Body image, the reminder of our overwhelming addiction to food as a society, and the insistence that we should be different. The amount of food that is thrust at people on a daily basis is constantly at war with the weight-loss tactics, healthy options, and otherwise digitally perfected image of what we should look like.

. . .

THINK ABOUT IT. Many of the great movie stars and iconic people of the seventies, eighties, and nineties are now getting up to their senior years. The people who are expected to adhere to body image the most are now in their fifties, or far beyond that. Yet, many of them still maintain an image, at least on camera, of being ageless. While we might not be held to those standards, they are the people that many people who are now seniors see. Those are the people that seniors are used to idolizing.

SENIORS, people over fifty, are becoming a lot more connected than seniors of the past. Thanks to social networks, cellphones and the internet in general, the connectivity seniors have is growing. While they did not grow up with this technology, they were able to watch it evolve. Therefore, a lot of seniors are involved in the same world as the younger generation. They see the same pictures, read the same stories and enjoy the same level of connectivity as the younger generation.

WHILE, for the most part, that is excellent, this also means that there is no filter. They see the same aging celebrities...and they still look great.

.   .   .

THEREFORE, seniors, at least at a subconscious level are presented with these warring sides of gluttony and beauty. Most people want to find some happy medium.

THE GOOD NEWS about Intermittent Fasting is that if you really need breakfast, or you need to eat something as soon as you get up, you can. Intermittent Fasting does not insist that you refrain from eating when you wake up. If you choose the morning to be the time that you eat, that is completely fine.

THE PROBLEM IS that you will have to go all day without eating. (We will get to the hangups with this a little later. *Spoiler* It has nothing to do with health. Again, it tests the endurance of the person who is fasting.

NOW, it is important, especially for Seniors or people over 50, that before starting any diet regiment, you should consult your doctor. There are some seniors that cannot fast, due to their medication or other health specifications. It is important to know this before you do anything to change your diet.

. . .

EVEN IF YOUR doctor gives the all-clear for you to start an Intermittent Fasting diet, you should remain under close supervision. Weight Loss, especially for seniors, is not a race and it is not a solo endeavor. Having a support system that ensures you are being taken care of and getting enough of what your body needs, is essential to success.

IS INTERMITTENT FASTING SAFE FOR SENIORS?

*Y*es. Intermittent Fasting is safe for seniors and can actually fit their natural desire for food. After all, as people get older, they tend to require less sustenance. While the choices that a person makes during this time is still essential to health, intermittent fasting can help seniors get into a routine that they enjoy.

STUDIES HAVE SHOWN that Intermittent Fasting can help people of all ages *lose weight, build muscle, boost their metabolism, lose fat, improve your memory, heal your body, and be more productive.* The reason this sounds like an infomercial is because many diets offer these promises. That doesn't mean they are wrong. In fact, there are studies that show this is more accurate for Intermittent Fasting than many other diets. However, ultimately, most diets that do anything make the person healthier. If you are healthier, you are going to feel a difference in these areas. You are going to lose weight and fat. You are going to build muscle. You are going to improve your memory, heal your body, and be more productive. That is simply the benefit of being a healthy individual. The diet that you choose is simply the vehicle that helps you get to those healthy results.

NOW, here are a few intriguing benefits of Intermittent Fasting that are not usually part of the weight-loss, fad diet speal:

INTERMITTENT FASTING CAN IMPROVE **insulin resistance**.

Intermittent Fasting can **protect against cognitive decline**.

Intermittent Fasting can **slow down the aging process**.

Intermittent Fasting can **fight cancer**.

YES, this is all true. There is scientific research that backs these testaments up and many of these benefits are specifically appealing to a senior audience.

. . .

ADDITIONALLY, Intermittent Fasting is good for seniors with specific health issues. (Be warned, some of these health issues seem like Intermittent Fasting would make it worse, but give it a chance.)

Diabetes:

Heart Health

Alzheimer's

- Reducing levels of insulin, which makes it easier for the body to use stored fat.
- Lowering blood sugars, blood pressure, and inflammation levels.
- Changing the expression of certain genes, which helps the body protect itself from disease as well as promoting longevity.
- Dramatically increases human growth hormone, or HGH, which helps the body utilize body fat and grow muscle.
- The body activates the healing process doctors call autophagy, which essentially means that the body digests or recycles old or damaged cell components.

Who Should NOT Try Intermittent Fasting?

- **You're pregnant:** Okay, so it is very possible that for seniors, or those over fifty, this is not a risk you are going to have to worry about. HOWEVER, on the off chance that you are pregnant over fifty, or you are thinking of partnering with a body that is pregnant, you do not want to try Intermittent Fasting while pregnant. When a woman is pregnant, her body is supplying nutrients for two lives. While the pregnant woman does not want to use this as a license to eat and she should maintain a healthy diet, it should not be a restrictive diet. Denying yourself food while pregnant is bad, both for the mother and the baby. Even people who fast for religious purposes do not mandate that pregnant women partake in the fast.

- **You have a history of an eating disorder:** Intermittent Fasting can be a trigger for an eating disorder. First, while the person is not eating, they can be plagued with a recurrence of the disorder, through which they do not eat. Second, when the person is no longer on the diet, they can dramatically overeat, which could cause the person's disorder to return. Of course, overeating is a possibility for anyone after they have finished the diet, but people who have a history of eating disorders are much more susceptible.

- **You are chronically stressed:** Stress can be affected by so many different things. Sometimes it is hard to decide whether you are doing something good for yourself, or not, because both reactions are stressful. Being unhealthy is stressful, both on your body and your mind. However, diet and exercise, especially for seniors who are thinking of trying Intermittent Fasting, is stressful too. This is why it is important to talk to your doctor to make sure that your stress will not be an issue for you, before you start any kind of life-changing diet.

- **You don't sleep well:** Changes in your diet, especially fasting does not help you sleep better. (At least, not at the beginning.) Once you get into a routine of a balanced diet and your body stops demanding food you do not need, people tend to sleep better. However, for seniors and everyone else, if you do not get sleep, you cannot function. Getting to the point where you are healthy and feel good might take longer than you should go without sleep. Therefore, if you already have an issue sleeping, you are not going to want to add insult to injury by fasting and losing more sleep than you do already.

HOW TO FAST INTERMITTENTLY

 *T*here are many ways to go about Intermittent Fasting. However, ultimately, fasting is fasting. The method you choose is specific to you. As it pertains to the length of time a person fasts, it is more of what you can handle. Admittedly, if you fast for longer periods of time, the weight loss is likely going to be quicker. After all, the longer your body has to rely on its stored fats, the more stored fats it uses up.

HOWEVER, when it comes to seniors, ESPECIALLY, there are many different factors to consider. Taking your pills, exercising, and your specific sustenance needs, all play a part in how long you should fast for.

. . .

THE ONE GOOD thing about Intermittent Fasting is that there are options. Whether you are working up to a higher fasting period or you are comfortable where you are is completely up to you. Regardless, if you are maintaining a healthy, balanced diet when you eat, you are going to be healthier. Even though the benefits might come faster or take a little longer, depending on the fasting time and dedication.

YET, the important thing is that you are doing the best you can. Any improvement is better than nothing at all.

1. Fast for 12 hours a day

Fortunately, this diet is simple to follow. Most of the fasting diets are but this 12 Hour Fasting diet is one of the easiest to follow. When you fast for 12 hours per day, you split your day in half. You pick a 12-hour fasting window every day. For that half of the day, whether it is the first half or the second half, you refrain from eating. All you drink is water, coffee (black), or tea (without anything in it). For the other twelve hours, you would be able to eat normally. However, you need to have a balanced breakfast.

The easiest way to do the 12-hour fast is to sleep for most of the fasting period. This may sound like cheating but it is not. (Especially if you are a person who likes to sit in front of the television and snack, this could be a big adjustment for you.)

A TIME PERIOD that many fasting participants have found is useful to them is to fast between 7 p.m. and 7 a.m. That means that your dinner would be finished before 7 p.m. and you would not be able to have any calories before 7 a.m.

THE IDEOLOGY:

FOR THIS FIRST IDEOLOGY, here is a wonderful revelation, from Plato, one of the most prolific historical thinkers: *"I fast for greater physical and mental efficiency."*

APPARENTLY, though, the Athenian philosopher was not the only person who was convinced that fasting was a gateway to better health and productivity. Here is the list of famous people who were quoted praising the benefits of fasting:

- **Benjamin Franklin**- To be fair, he weighed in on almost everything.

- **Hippocrates**-The most notable of the three fathers of Western medicine. (Specifically, he believed in starving sickness.)
- **Mark Twain**- Twain also believed that starving sickness was often better than medication.
- **Plutarch**- He was a Greek biographer and moralist that would rather people use fasting before medication. The interesting thing about Plutarch having this opinion is that he was tasked with recording the lives of the people around him. Therefore, he was able to have a first-hand account of what people were going through and what remedies were most successful. (Granted, the medicine they had in Ancient Greece was likely not as effective as today. Yet, he is not the first, nor the last influential person to publicly promote this belief.)

THE TAKEAWAY from sharing this is to explain that fasting is not new and it is not only part of modern religious practices. It is something that is difficult but it has its rewards. Even if a person only fasts for a little while, it is still better than succumbing to your every urge. Research shows that after twelve hours, your body starts burning fat, as opposed to burning glycogen. (This is a body chemical composition that burns sugar but this is still essential to be healthier.) The benefits of fasting are supposed to start after doing start and ramp up between ten and fourteen hours, so twelve is a good midway point, especially if you are starting out.

- **Brain Health:** Our brain is an essential part of our cognizance. Psychology is even finding that people with certain personalities and a predisposition to different illnesses can be predicted by the shape of a person's brain. Crazy, right?

HOWEVER, this information is only a fraction of the known importance of a person's brain. Therefore, it makes sense to ensure the brain is happy and healthy. Science suggests that reducing caloric intake will help brain functionality and aging. This belief causes doctors to hypothesize that caloric restriction and Intermittent Fasting will reduce the development and progression of Alzheimer's.

- **Extreme Detox:** Everything your body does burns energy. Repairing itself, burning fat, and detoxing itself all takes energy. The problem is many of us continually have is that we do not allow our bodies time to detox older, stored fat. Instead, we keep eating, so our body has to constantly try to mitigate any immediate threat from fresh toxins. This adds to the sludge that our body has to wade through in order to function. If we fast (even for a twelve-hour period) it gives our body a chance to detox some of the older, stored fats that have built up. Of course, the longer you fast, the better off your body will be (in this regard). Yet, the benefits are seen during a twelve-hour fast.

- **Reduces Inflammation:** This is another benefit for people who fall into the senior's age-range. Even if seniors are in good shape, there is a risk of serious inflammation. The risk is due to medical issues, old injuries, and other common problems that seniors face. Research has shown that fasting activates the NRF2 Pathway. Recently, this pathway has been linked to helping humans overcome many degenerative afflictions that are common among seniors.

Will Cole, D.C., a functional medicine expert and

best-selling author of Ketotarian said, ""Since some of the benefits of fasting include reduced inflammation, loading up on junk food during your eating window can perpetuate this inflammation. And with inflammation being the underlying contributing factor in almost all modern-day health problems, this is something you definitely want to keep under control."

Issues with the 12-Hour Diet:

Stress Levels are Boosted During Fasting

Stress levels are higher during fasting because you are putting your body in an uncomfortable situation. Fasting, whether it is for twelve hours or twenty-four hours is hard. Your body is not used to fasting at all; most of us are trained to eat when our body tells us we are hungry. Thus, to go against that is an issue that makes our body react. This reaction results in higher stress levels.

This makes Intermittent Fasting difficult, for any length of time, for people with anxiety, a cardiac history, or anything that can be stress-induced.

However, that does not mean that everyone with a cardiac history, an issue with anxiety, or otherwise cannot participate in Intermittent Fasting. (This is especially true for people who are trying out twelve-hour fasting because it is not a prolonged time period.) All this means is that you should be aware of it. Understanding your body is one of the best ways to get healthy; period. You need to listen to what your body is telling you and decide accordingly. If you are feeling too stressed, or your body does not seem to be handling prolonged periods of fasting, try shorter intervals and talk to your doctor.

Binge Eating

Unfortunately, it is common for people to break their fast, either for the day or all together and binge-eat. Even with only fasting for twelve hours, it is possible to fall into the trap of feeling like you must eat a quick, likely unhealthy meal to *get your sugar back up* or something similar. While this does not negate your fasting time, it is not a healthy move. A quick sugar rush might make your body feel better initially. Yet, relying on sugar and quick sustenance fixes is not good for anyone in the long-term.

Fasting for 16 hours or the 16/8 Fasting Option or the Leangains diet

This is the most common form of Intermittent Fasting because it fits nicely into most people's schedules (and can often give them some time for themselves, when they would otherwise be busy eating). This diet requires men to fast for 16 hours a day, and women to fast for at least 14 hours per day. This leaves an eight-hour eating window for men and a ten-hour eating window for women. (Women can choose to fast for the full 16 hours but some women believe their hormones might go awry if they do.)

. . .

THIS IS a step up from the 12 hour diet, because it is longer. This fasting period is challenging but it is fairly convenient and gives the body a little extra time to use that stored fat as energy before glucose is returned to the system. This is a great option if you did not see any improvement from trying out a 12-hour diet. Remember, work your way up so you do not overwhelm your system.

WHILE THE TIME period is not ironclad, for most participants of this method of Intermittent Fasting, people finish their evening meal by 8 p.m. The next day, they wake up and go about their business without eating until noon. After that, the participant has until 8 p.m. that evening to get their recommended amount of daily carbs.

ONE EXTREMELY INTERESTING study that was done on mice indicated that the group that was limited to the eight-hour feeding window were protected them from obesity, inflammation, diabetes, and liver disease, better than those that ate whenever they wanted. The findings were despite the time-restricted mice eating the same number of calories as mice that ate at will throughout the day.

. . .

The Ideology:

The ideology behind this extremely popular Intermittent Fasting method is less about what you eat and more about the time you give your body in a fasting state. Of course, it is more beneficial to eat healthy but the point of this method is more about time than the consumption. Here are the benefits to this diet:

- **Long-Term Weight Loss Solution:** Yes, this method does help participants lose weight and they do not have to count calories to do it. This is a non-conventional method of weight loss that is still rising in its popularity but there are many things about this particular Intermittent Fasting method that is promising. One highly regarded benefit is that this method is highly conducive to transitioning into a lifestyle. For this method, if it is followed conventionally, with participants only eating between noon and eight at night, there is a limited time during the day when food is restricted. Once twelve o'clock hits, fasting is finished and they have eight hours to do what they want. (But they still get the health benefits of the diet.)

- **Helps People Who Are Pre-Diabeitic:** Pre-Diabeties affects 84.1 million Americans, according to a report by the CDC. This means that within five years, if the people diagnosed pre-diabetic, do not diet and exercise, changing their lifestyle completely, they will have Type 2 Diabetes. There are two reasons this method of Intermittent Fasting works so well to ward off this terrible disease. First, this is a diet that people with unhealthy eating habits can lean into. The fact that they do not have restrictions on their diet, during their eight hour period makes it easier for pre-diabetics to make progress without turning their whole world upside down.

The second reason this method works so well is that research shows that this diet can restore insulin secretion and promote the generation of new insulin-producing cells. Even more promising, is that the generation of new cells works for both Type 1 and Type 2 Diabetes, at least in mice. If this information is true for humans, though it could open a whole new door for people who are born with the terrible disease.

- **Can Slow Down the Aging Process:** The aging process is hindered by a robust mitochondria. The mitochondria is the powersource for cells and is responsible for putting out mitochondrial stress responses. This helps your body deal with stress better and thus, helps the aging process slow down. This is also theorized to help fight against and prevent other diseases.

- **Helps Sync Circadian Rhythm:** This benefit has to do with your internal clock. Basically, Intermittent Fasting helps to reset your internal clock and align it with your circadian rhythm. This helps your body to understand what is needed at what time. Being in sync with your circadian rhythm is also theorized to help fight and prevent metabolic diseases.

Issues with the 16:8 Intermittent Fasting Method:

Does Not Teach a Healthy Diet:

A lot of the issues with this diet stem from the idea that even though it is possible to lose weight with this method of Intermittent Fasting, is it really healthy? Yes, the diet encourages people to eat healthy but really, there is no actual direction. As long as the person keeps to only eating eight hours per day, research shows that they will reap at least some of the benefits of Intermittent Fasting, even if they do not change their eating habits. This is not good for long-term health. Even if people lose weight while working on this Intermittent Fasting method, their health can still suffer, if they do not eat a balanced diet.

Lack of Sufficient Research:

There is a lot of questions of not whether this is sustainable, but rather, if it should be sustainable. There is a lack of sufficient research to tell anyone if this method is good or bad for people. Ultimately, everything that is known is theorized and there is no concrete evidence of how this method of weight loss will affect people in the future. Therefore, everything that is happening, good and bad, is still theory. There are no true hardened facts. Even the people who have conducted studies on the subject have said that there is still a lot of room for study and observation. Unfortunately, a lot of that will only come with time.

3. Fasting for 2 Days a Week

This diet is also referred to as the 5:2 diet. Basically, this means that the participant eats standard amounts of **healthful** food for 5 days and reduces their calorie intake on the other 2 days. This, again, is a little different for men and women, if they choose. During the two days of fasting, men are advised to consume 600 calories. Women are advised to consume 500 calories.

PEOPLE WHO PARTAKE in this method of Intermittent Fasting usually separate their fasting days, to different portions of the week. That way, they can give their bodies a break.

AN EXAMPLE WOULD BE if they fast on Monday and Thursday, then the person would eat as they normally would, three healthy meals on the remaining days.

ADDITIONALLY, with this method of Intermittent Fasting, there should be at least one day between the two fasting days. This practice will help avoid overwhelming their system.

EVEN THOUGH THE amount of calories consumed on fast days are obnoxiously small, there is no set time period. They are fasting all day, so they have the opportunity to possibly curb their hunger with mini snacks before it gets to be an issue.

· · ·

UNFORTUNATELY, though, there is very little research done on this specific method. Most of the studies are minor, with a limited number of participants. However, there has been a lot of different benefits found throughout the studies that were conducted.

THE IDEOLOGY:

The ideology behind the 5:2 diet, or the "Fast Diet" is that the benefits of Intermittent Fasting can be achieved, even without fasting like crazy. Even though the two days per week probably are not the most pleasant in the world, practitioners of this diet find it easier than only having more fasting to look forward to in the morning. Here are the benefits that are found to be associated with the 5:2 Intermittent Fasting diet:

- **Protection From Disease:** Much like the other Intermittent Fasting methods, the 5:2 diet is alleged to help protect participants from diseases. It is prone to helping participants who are teetering on the edge of diabetes, as well as those who have a possibility of Dementia and Alzheimers. Fasting in general helps defend against and prevent a plethora of different conditions but this one is a method specific to cognitive degeneration ailments. Plus, these methods are known to aid in resisting the effects of aging.

- **Increased Lifespan:** It is no secret that eating less (and eating healthier) will lead to a longer natural lifespan. Yet, the sheer amount of benefits that go beyond weight loss is staggering. While there has not been a lot of research that specifically targets the 5:2 Intermittent Fasting diet, the evidence that is collected paints a clear picture of health benefits that, as far as we know it, will lead to an increased lifespan and possibly, cures for diseases that plague people all over the world.

Issues with the 5:2 Intermittent Fasting Method:

Even though this might be a more comfortable fasting experience, at least five days out of the week, when you aren't fasting, the back and forth certainly seems like it is asking a lot from the body. The body, as well as the mind, likes to have a schedule that works with its internal clock. Getting up, going to bed, and eating are three of the main constants that a body looks for in a schedule. However, this particular method seems to have issues that toy with every aspect of scheduling stability.

Difficulty Sleeping

One of the main issues with this particular method of Intermittent Fasting is that people have a hard time sleeping. However, this does make sense, as the inconsistency of this method is sure to disturb your internal clock. Fasting is a big enough change but even if you consciously know when you are going to be fasting, your body is worried about it, because there is no flow. If you fast every day, your body can settle into a routine. However, when it gets to be every other day, twice a week, or once a week, your body becomes riddled with anxiety. This keeps you up at night.

Dehydration

Often, when people do not eat, they also forget to drink. Since this is not an every-day fast, it is sometimes difficult for participants to remember to drink more water on their fast days. If you are doing this twice a week, it will add up and before too long, it will become a problem. As a senior, you do not want to get too dehydrated or that could have a domino effect for other medical conditions. Here are a few early warning signs of dehydration to keep an eye out for:

- Dark Urine
- Changes in Skin: Tone, Temperature, or Texture

- Dry or Sticky Mouth
- Constipation
- Extreme Hunger Pains
- Headache
- Fatigue
- Nausea
- Mood Swings

IT WILL NEVER HURT to drink more water, so if you notice these symptoms, try quenching your thirst. Yet, if the symptoms worsen or do not go away, make sure to see a doctor immediately.

Daytime Sleepiness

Another common side effect of 5:2 Intermittent Fasting is daytime sleepiness. This could be extremely dangerous for people of any age, but specifically seniors. Since this messes up your internal clock, participants feel tired when they are supposed to be awake and unable to go to sleep when they are supposed to be tired. Daytime Sleepiness, especially if the person gives into it, can lead to a revolving door of an unhealthy sleeping schedule that could possibly outlast the fast itself.

ULTIMATELY, the 5:2 Intermittent Fasting method is not recommended for seniors. While many of the benefits are directed at seniors, a lot of the side effects could trigger a host of issues for seniors.

4. A weekly 24-hour fast

This is an interesting fast. It takes a lot of strength, endurance, and before trying it, you should probably have medical clearance. This is the 24-hour Intermittent Fasting diet. When a person is on this diet, all they can have for twenty-four hours at a time is water, teas, and calorie-free drinks. This can be done for one or two days per week. (It is not recommended for more than that.)

A LOT of people who take part in this diet find that fasting from breakfast to breakfast or lunch to lunch is a good way to help stave off the hunger and you have something in your stomach each day, just not during a twenty-four hour period.

ONCE THE TWENTY-FOUR hours is up, though, participants should eat normally, for at least one day before returning to a fasted state. This diet reduces a person's calorie intake significantly but it does not deny participants any specific foods on non-fast days. This means that the person is able to eat whatever they want throughout the course of the non-fast days. Although, it is recommended that a person eat a balanced diet.

· · ·

A 24-HOUR FAST IS DIFFICULT. There is no way around it and seniors are heavily cautioned against this difficult fast. It is reported that this type of fast causes extreme fatigue, headaches, and often, irritability. It is stated that many people report these side effects lessening significantly over time. Yet, it can take a while for the body to adjust to this new pattern of eating. Many people are not able to handle this extreme fast and some people, seniors specifically, shouldn't push it with this extreme form of fasting.

FOR ANYONE TRYING this type of fast, it is important to note that to be successful, it is advised that you try a 12-hour or 16-hour fast first. If that is successful and you feel the need to try a 24-hour fast, then you can. However, going into something like that as a green faster could be immensely uncomfortable.

THE IDEOLOGY:

THERE ARE some major benefits to this type of fasting. Even though this is an extremely difficult fasting method, the hard work might be worth it. After all, this is only a once or twice per week endeavor. That is something that you are going to have to decide for yourself.

HERE ARE the different benefits that are theorized to be a result of 24-hour fasting:

- **Promotes Blood Sugar Control:** Studies have found evidence that fasting may improve blood sugar control. While this is good for anyone, especially with the high rate of pre-diabetes affecting Americans, this is also a benefit for those who have diabetes. The reason this is theorized to be so successful is that 24-hour fasting decreases a person's insulin resistance. When our body is more sensitive to insulin, glucose is able to travel through a person's bloodstream and reach your cells, where they can be used for energy with a greater level of ease.

- **May Enhance Heart Health:** Studies have shown that different functions of heart health are greatly improved by 24-hour fasting. These functions include the stabilization of:

- Blood Pressure
- Triglycerides
- Cholesterol Levels

IT IS KNOWN that opting for a better diet and changing your lifestyle is the best way to combat the risk of heart disease and other cardiac ailments. However, these result are not necessarily because people are eating healthier; it is just because they are eating less per week.

Some research has found that incorporating fasting into your routine may be especially beneficial when it comes to heart health.

- **Increases Growth Hormone Secretion:** While an increase in secretion is usually a bad thing, increasing growth hormone secretion is essential for healthy living. Human Growth Hormone (unceremoniously also known as HGH) is a protein that is vital for (you guessed it) growth. However, this hormone and other hormones like it are also responsible for a healthy metabolism, promoting weight loss, and helping create muscle strength.
- **May Aid in Cancer Prevention and Increase the Effectiveness of Chemotherapy:** It is understandable that the last thing a person may want to do

while undergoing Chemotherapy is fast. After all, Chemo messes with so much of your body, a patient often wants to salvage every normal feeling and luxury they can. However, there are a few studies that have indicated fasting may benefit the treatment and prevention of cancer.

Unfortunately, the studies that have to do with this particular benefit are still in their infancy. It could be some time before any truly useful information is garnered. Nevertheless, the studies that were conducted are promising and scientists are hopeful that this information is the beginning of a breakthrough with cancer research.

ISSUES WITH 24-HOUR INTERMITTENT FASTING:

The longer a person fasts, the more complicated living normal life through fasting can be. Of course, there are usually ways around most issues but seniors need to be very careful. Unfortunately, a lot of the issues that can be helped by fasting, allegedly, can also be made worse by the lack of food.

Taking Medication that Requires Food:

Fasting is not easy. Fasting for any length of time, any amount during the week has its struggles. However, it is often extremely challenged when it comes to 24-hour fasting sessions. When you go an entire day without food, there are many more issues that arise besides hunger and a headache. One of the most prominent issues is that of medication. If you take medication, which many seniors do, a lot of the medication is to be taken with food. This is mandatory, or your body could have severe reactions. If this is the case, depending on the times your medicine needs to be taken, 24-hour fasting might not be for you at all.

GRANTED, it is usually possible to take medication with food, while still adhering to your fast if you only take the medication once per day. Remember, many people start their fast after breakfast one day and eat lunch on the following day. Your 24-hour fast does not have to fit into a traditional day. Time is time and your body will fast the same regardless of when you start or finish.

IF YOU DO THIS THOUGH, you are going to want to take your medication on day one with your last meal of the day. Then, the following day, you are going to want to take your medicine with the first meal after your fast.

Previous Medical Conditions:

Fasting for 24-hours will not kill you. You will not starve within a day without food. It will be uncomfortable and it will not be easy but you will not succumb to starvation. However, if you have a previous medical condition, such as diabetes, cardiac issues, anxiety, or a history of any food-related disorder, you should think twice about fasting for 24-hours. Depending on medical involvement and your specific history, you might be advised not to fast at all. Yet, even if you can fast, there is a big difference in fasting for 12 and 16 hours, opposed to not eating for 24-hours. Therefore, seniors and anyone else with prior medical conditions should talk to their doctor and find out what is appropriate for them, specifically.

THE ODD THING about fasting is that it seems to have long-term benefits, that first challenge short-term survivability; or comfortability, at the very least. While a lot of younger people can endure the side effects of fasting, seniors need to be careful. While that doesn't mean that seniors should avoid fasting. Yet, they should be cautious when they are fasting. It can be difficult to know when you are overdoing it until you have overdone it. This goes for people of all ages. Thus, it is important to stay connected with your body and with your doctor, when you are attempting any type of lifestyle change.

Meal Skipping

At first glance the "meal skipping" diet seems to

be Intermittent Fasting with training wheels. This approach to weight loss is extremely flexible and is known for being good for beginners. With this approach, a person eats normal (hopefully healthy) meals and occasionally purposefully skips a meal. The meal that is skipped does not really matter, because you are going through the same basic period of time without eating.

WITH THIS MORE WHIMSICAL METHOD, participants are able to decide which meals to skip, so that the meal they miss does not interrupt anything important. Additionally, having the ability to decide which meal to skip can be a time-saver. For instance, if you do not stop for lunch, you gain not only the time you would be eating but the cool down and ramp-up period of going away and coming back to whatever you are doing.

RESEARCHERS SAY that Meal Skipping going to be most successful when participants are able to accurately respond to their body's hunger signals. In addition to eating when they are hungry and skipping meals when they are not hungry, this also means that the person is drinking enough water and getting enough activity. This way, they are not mistaking another desire, such as thirst or the body's response to complacency as hunger. That will likely only add insult to injury.

The Ideology:

A MEAL NOT EATEN, as long as you only eat the next meal like you normally would, is a reduction in calories. If a person systematically reduces their calorie intake, they will lose weight and see the benefits of their efforts. While, this is not exactly fasting, because the time frame isn't long enough, it does help people decide whether or not they want to dive into fasting for a long period of time.

- **Can Feel More Natural:** People skip meals all the time. Whether they are working late, not feeling well, or just get busy and time gets away from the, most people have skipped a meal here and there. That is part of what makes this type of "fasting" seem more natural. With this type of fasting, you are not held to a schedule. It can be decided instantly and it doesn't interfere with medication or plans. Plus, if you do end up eating, there is no guilt, because you have no actual plan. You aren't doing anything wrong or against your diet. After all, there is always the next meal.

- **Offers a Trial Period of Sorts:** There seems to be a trial period for nearly everything. The idea of a trial period is a non-committal agreement with a service that lets you see if you want to commit to the full service. Meal Skipping is kind of like the trial period for Intermittent Fasting. If you skip a meal, see how you feel. If you skip meals consistently, see if there is an improvement, or if there is an issue. This way, you have a better understanding of what to tell the doctor, should you decide to talk about graduating to a full-scale Intermittent Fasting method.

- **Can Help You Lose Weight:** Even though this is not a full fasting method, you can still lose weight. If you are diligent about skipping meals on a consistent basis and make an effort to be healthier when you do eat, there is a possibility that you will start to lose weight. This might not be as quick but if you are worried about the adverse effects of actual Intermittent Fasting, this is a positive and less stressful alternative.

Issues with Meal Skipping:

The fact that Meal Skipping is not quite Intermittent Fasting poses some issues. First and foremost, people using this method are fasting without getting nearly the amount of benefits. After all, whether you miss one meal or three meals, you are still hungry and you likely still have a headache but the difference in benefits between one and two or three meals is staggering.

There is No Direction

Skipping meals does have benefits and could be a great pre-game for actual Intermittent Fasting. Yet, for long-term use, there is no direction. Even though part of the allure for this method is that it is far less taxing and more whimsical than other fasting tactics, there is no actual direction. People are left to figure it all out by themselves, which can sometimes do more harm than good.

Most Fasting Benefits Are Not Available with this Method :

It is common sense that if you eat less, especially when it comes to calories, you will lose weight. This is especially true if you maintain healthy eating habits throughout the rest of the week. Although, the weight loss is a slow process and could be discouraging. Furthermore, the rest of the health benefits that are theoretically contributed to fasting does not apply. After all, this method is not really fasting. It is simply skipping a meal.

ULTIMATELY, Meal Skipping is good for people who wish to test the water with fasting, without jumping into a full fasting regimen. This is a good way to tell how you are going to feel and if any issues will arise but this is not recommended for long-term dieting.

6. The Warrior Diet

While Meal Skipping is not quite there, the Warrior Diet is the over-achiever version of Intermittent Fasting. The Warrior Diet demands that participants eat very little for 20 hours, every day. Although, water is still encouraged, along with a few tiny servings of raw fruit, and vegetables. Once the 20-hour fasting window is over, the participant is able to eat one large meal. This is kind of a last-resort type of Intermittent Fasting. It is certainly not something that people just wake up one day and start doing. It is hard, primarily because it is exactly the opposite of what most of us were taught about eating. Forget about tiny meals and consistent protein, this diet exclaims that it is good for the body for people to eat at night.

BELIEVERS of the Warrior Diet argue that humans are naturally nocturnal eaters. Their claim is that eating at night enables the body to gain nutrients in line with its circadian rhythms.

ALTHOUGH, that is kind of hard to believe. Unless you're eating a Thanksgiving Dinner before going to bed, most people are going to be up all night after one big meal. During this one meal, people are expected to eat vegetables, proteins, and healthy fats. They should also include some carbohydrates.

THERE IS ALSO a risk that people on this diet will not eat enough nutrients, such as fiber. This can increase the risk of cancer and have an adverse effect on digestive and immune health.

THE IDEOLOGY:

THE IDEOLOGY behind this method of fasting is odd. There is not a lot of information to back up the claims of the Warrior Diet. In fact, most research would caution against it. Yet, here are the benefits that this diet claims to hold:

- **Effective Weight Loss:** Obviously, weight loss is a big part of why people diet.

However, the amount of weight loss possible through the Warrior Diet is significant. There are two main reasons for this. The first, is that the participant is only eating one meal per day. There is only so much we can eat at one time. Therefore, there is only so much consumption possible. The second reason is the majority of the twenty hours out of the day is spent using stored fat as fuel instead of glucose. Even if you get a little bit of exercise each day while on this diet, you are expediting the fat burning process exponentially.

- **Low Blood Pressure:** Generally, if you lose weight, you are going to have lower blood pressure. That is just how it works. The more fat is burned, the easier the blood flows through your veins and thus, the lower the pressure. However, with the intense amount of fat that is burned each day while on the Warrior Diet helps that process along, which actually makes it easier for fat to flow to the cells and are used for fuel. It is interesting how all of these seemingly unrelated pieces fit together so nicely.
- **Helps Build and Maintain Muscle Mass:** It is a common misconception that fasting

breaks down muscle mass. In fact, it preserves and increases it while your body breaks down stored fat in its time of need. This is important for seniors because eventually, muscle mass will begin to break down on its own. When the body starts to wear out, (you know, a long, long time from now,) your muscle mass will deplete. This is why falling is such a common risk for seniors. Their body's muscles are not what they used to be and so it is harder to keep upright. The good news is, if a senior works to continue building and preserving muscle mass, the effects of depletion will be slowed significantly.

Issues with the Warrior Diet:

This diet is not a simple diet to follow or to complete. Until your body gets used to the new feeding and fasting schedule, every day will be a challenge. Now, the question is, will that challenge be worth it in the end? You have already read the theorized benefits, now here are the issues with the Warrior Diet:

There is a high dropout rate:

It does make sense that something with the name "the Warrior Diet" wasn't going to be an easy accomplishment. As a senior, though, you might want to try this diet just so you can prove that you can do it. However, there are legitimate concerns with the Warrior Diet, for seniors and for everybody else. Going twenty hours every day with barely any food is extremely difficult. People reportedly have headaches, dizziness, fatigue, irritability, and trouble sleeping. Even though every fasting method is a big change to a person's lifestyle, the Warrior Diet is one of the most severe. Regardless of whether you have fasted successfully before or not, this is a big adjustment.

There is not a lot of research that backs the claims of the die hard Warrior Diet Fans:

This is a big deal because something smells fishy with this diet. Despite the fact that this is considered a real Intermittent Fasting method, there is even less information about it then the other methods. While none of the other methods are overly researched, this one is strange, right from the get-go. Most authorities claim that having a large meal in the evening is bad for your metabolism and sleep cycle. Most of the other Intermittent Fasting methods begrudgingly agree. The Warrior Diet is the only one that gets in the face of this commonly-known belief and admittedly denies it's authority. Then, to top it all off, there are no really good studies that support this method's claims. The only thing we are sure of, is that the Warrior Diet, if it can be stuck to, is a good way to lose weight. Otherwise, people do not really have any idea how true the benefits really are.

It's adverse effects seem to negate a lot of the positive benefits a participant hopes for:

Each fasting method has a possibility of adverse effects. However, this specific method of fasting has a negative effect for nearly every positive benefit. While other fasting methods boast that participants are usually full of energy, especially in the middle of their fast, the effects of this method says people complain of low energy. Plus, due to the extreme nature of this period of fasting, it is difficult for people with diabetes or other preexisting conditions to get through the initial stages. A lot of the time, their ailments make it difficult, sometimes even dangerous for people to persevere, to reap the benefits that fasting awards.

IN SUMMATION, the Warrior Diet does obviously work for some people. However, any senior, or otherwise, who wishes to try it should be careful. Make sure you do your own research, work your way up to a twenty-hour, daily fast, and make sure you know what you are doing before you start this fasting method. The most important thing is if something starts to feel off, go to the doctor. Do not brush it off. There is discomfort because you are fasting and then there is a potentially life-threatening issue. You will know the difference if you listen to your body.

A STEP BY STEP BREAKDOWN OF
THE 16:8 METHOD

$\mathcal{T}$he 16:8 Intermittent Fasting method is a favorite among most people who are trying to get into a healthy routine through this diet. This is a safe diet for the majority of seniors and people tend to be able to lock into this diet much easier, making it more conducive to a lifestyle change.

HERE ARE the things you need to consider for a day in the life of what is possible for a typical 16:8 Intermittent Fasting Day:

Figure Out a Timeline:

First, you need to decide when you are going to start your fasting. This could depend on your medication schedule, your sleep schedule, and your hunger schedule. Remember, you want to make this diet as convenient as possible for you. That way, there is less of a chance that you are going to be tempted to cheat or break your fast early.

BASICALLY, you have to ask yourself, are you a morning person, or a night person? If you are a night snacker, you might want to be done with your fast in the afternoon, so you can eat at night without breaking your fast.

ALTHOUGH, if you are a person that has to eat as soon as their feet hit the floor, you are going to want to make breakfast the first meal that breaks your fast.

ALSO, remember that is okay to switch the timeline around a little. Try both a morning fast and an evening fast. See which one works better for you. This is not a one-size fits all diet. That is why there are so many different methods. Depending on your goals and your personal preferences, seniors have plenty of options to choose from when it comes to Intermittent Fasting.

Figure Out a Workout Schedule:

GETTING MOVING and working out is a great way to

get healthy and help stave off the side effects of Intermittent Fasting. However, before you can do this, you have a few decisions to make.

First: What are you going to do?

When people think of exercise, more often than not, adults think about going to a gym. An image of a sweaty, muscled person on some kind of gym equipment comes to mind. For many of us, this is not an appealing image. So, if you are not going to do that, what are you going to do?

INSTEAD OF THINKING about traditional exercise, think about physical things you enjoy doing. Do you enjoy yoga? Do you like to play sports? Do you like to dance?

THINK of something physical that you like to do and find a way to do it. Exercise doesn't have to be confined to a gym unless you want it to be. If you cannot find a group to do something you want to do, create the group yourself. Get your friends together and go to a local park, or community center.

THE GOOD THING about having this freedom is that there is always a way. Even if you have to get creative, getting the exercise you need can be fun and doesn't have to break the bank. Sometimes, it just requires a little enginuity.

SECOND: Do you plan to exercise while fasting or during your non-fasting hours?

Science states that this is essentially up to the person who is exercising. While seniors are cautioned about the possible risks of exercising while in a fasted state, it does work for some people. Therefore, it is still a question that everyone should contemplate.

DO NOT OVERDO it but if you feel sluggish while exercising during your fasting hours, perhaps it is a good idea to give it a try. Obviously, you should watch yourself carefully but if you find it works for you, there are benefits to working out in a fasting state.

HOWEVER, if you do not think that is for you, that is fine as well. As long as you get up and get moving, somehow, at some point during the day, you are doing good.

THIRD: How often do you plan to work out?

Working out usually becomes a regimented thing. We might not intend for it to be but if you plan to stick to it, you need to make it a part of your schedule. So, how often are you planning to work out? Ideally, you want to have some kind of movement every day. It doesn't have to be a full-blown workout but it should be enough to get your blood pumping. Fortunately, exactly what you do every day does not have to be the same thing. Varying your workout, both by intensity and what you are doing to workout is a good way to keep everything fresh. Keeping it fun will help you get to a point where you look forward to it. It is no fun to do the same thing every day, so you want to mix it up. Life should be fun, so find a way to enjoy everything you do.

REWARD YOURSELF WITHOUT FOOD:

IT IS a common human nature trait to want to reward ourselves after we do a good job. Whether the good job was done at work, at home, through dieting, or on an un-edible project, the reward that many settle for is food. Almost everything revolves around food. When we are kids, we go for ice cream for a treat, or we get a candy bar. When we are an adult, to commemorate accomplishments, we go to dinner. When dieting, we reward ourselves for a week of following a diet with exactly what we spent all week staying away from.

So, much like a lot of other areas of a successful Intermittent Fasting experience, we need to turn the tables on the conventions we have grown up with. Now, that doesn't mean that you don't reward yourself. That's no fun. Instead, you need to find rewards that are enjoyable but not consumable. Instead of eating something, do something fun. Do something for yourself. Instead of eating your reward, make a memory. Spend time doing something you enjoy. Try something that you have always wanted to try. Take time and about the same amount of money you would spend on a meal and make it into an experience.

THE COOL THING about doing this, instead of settling for a meal, besides not eating, is that you are expanding your interests. The more you do this, the more inspired you will become. Instead of looking forward to food, soon, you will start to look forward to having fun and doing things for yourself.

MENU

The menu for the day is the most important part

as, regardless of what you're level of fitness is, you still like food. The affinity for sustenance is not going anywhere. By fasting and dieting, you are simply learning to control your body and make it work for you.

THAT MEANS, whether you like it or not, you are always going to look forward to meal time. So, here are three sample meal days by Mind, Body, Green:

EARLY EATING **window**

8 a.m.: Egg and Veggies (scrambled)
12 p.m.: Apple and Almond Butter
4 p.m.: Chicken and Veggie Stir Fry
Evening: Decaf Tea

MIDDAY EATING WINDOW

Morning: Black Coffee or Tea
11 a.m.: Banana and Peanut Butter Smoothie
2 p.m.: Avocado Toast with Pistachios
4 p.m.: Dark-Chocolate-Covered Almonds
6 p.m.: Turkey Meatballs and Tomato Sauce over Whole Wheat (or Zucchini Noodle) Pasta

LATE EATING WINDOW

Morning: Black Coffee or Tea
1 p.m.: Blackberry Chia Pudding
4 p.m.: Carrots and Hummus or Guacamole
9 p.m.: Grilled Salmon, Vegetables, and Quinoa

OF COURSE, these are super healthy options and while the meals go well together anything on this list is something that can be had, regardless of when your eating window is. However, it can be helpful to see different options, that many people may not even know exist!

THINGS TO KEEP IN MIND WHEN INTERMITTENT FASTING AS A SENIOR

*E*verybody is different. There are many people in this world. There are many different reasons why people should and should not take part in different activities. Remember, Intermittent Fasting is a lifestyle change. Even though it is good for you, there are certain people, with specific health issues that need to be more conscious of their fasting plans than others.

IT IS ALWAYS important to speak with your doctor before doing anything drastic to your diet and/or exercise regimen. Even after you are given the okay for this diet though, it is incredibly important to keep your doctors apprised of your progress. This is a big step for anyone but for seniors, it is even more important that they are able to be under the watchful eye of a professional.

THE GOOD NEWS IS, most doctors are going to be supportive of this change. If you are truly committed to Intermittent Fasting, you are committing to a major change in your lifestyle.

Do Not Use Poor Health as an Excuse

Yes, this book is totally calling you out. People do their best to stay within their comfort zone. It is natural. Remember, the path of least resistance is always going to look the brightest because your mind spit-shines it up to be appealing. Unfortunately, the easiest way is not always the best way, even if it is the most appealing. Therefore, it is important to keep

Risks of Intermittent Fasting for Seniors

Of course, there are risks. If there is no risk in what you are doing, you either aren't doing very much or your information is flawed. Everything has a risk. As a senior, especially, the risks for everything seem to be greater. This is an even greater challenge for seniors who are currently unhealthy.

THE REASON THIS IS IMPORTANT, though, is because even if there are risks involved, there is also a reward to be gained.

. . .

EVEN STILL, while Intermittent Fasting can drastically improve and elongate your life, for that to happen, you need to be aware of the risks as well as the benefits. Here is a list of the risks that are specific to Seniors who are thinking about Intermittent Fasting:

Disruptive Sleep Patterns

When people get older, they often do not need a lot of sleep. Yet, that does not mean that seniors can get away without sleeping or having disruptive sleep patterns. While Intermittent Fasting offers a lot of long-term benefits, one of the side effects that often plagues seniors is disruptive sleep patterns. This is worse for seniors than it is for other people because without sleep, it is hard to function. While for a younger person, not getting enough sleep is generally annoying, not getting enough sleep for seniors could lead to an emergency. Seniors who have continuously disrupted sleep can fall easier or fall asleep suddenly, causing a dangerous situation.

Dehydration

Intermittent Fasting can lead to dehydration, particularly for seniors, because for many people, food is the normal association of drink. When a person is not eating, they may simply forget to drink anything and that could lead to dehydration. Seniors are much more susceptible to dehydration because of aches, pains, and other medical conditions. Plus, if a senior lives alone, they may not have anyone who checks up on them every day, so they might not realize they are dehydrated until it becomes a serious situation. To remedy this, drink water throughout the day. A good number to stick to is three liters of water per day.

Anxiety

Anxiety can become a major problem for those who are trying any of the Intermittent Fasting methods. The reason is such a drastic change to the way a person eats is stressful to the body. That stress is compounded by the normal, everyday stress that people have, throughout their daily lives. The combination of this, for anyone can be difficult to handle, at least for a little while. However, with seniors, there is always the risk of anxiety triggering other medical issues. That is why anyone with heart problems or other conditions that are worsened by stress needs to see a doctor and get medical clearance before starting any Intermittent Fasting Method.

ADDITIONALLY, even after being cleared initially, it is important to keep your doctor apprised of your progress, your struggles and anything else that is going on.

Do Not Drink a lot of Alcohol

. . .

WHEN PEOPLE ARE FASTING, they should not drink a lot of alcohol. When people are in the middle of a fast, they should not drink any alcohol. It breaks a fast. (Yes, even if you leave out the lime.) Therefore, that leaves a limited amount of time for someone to enjoy a large quantity of alcohol. However, there are more reasons that alcohol is not the best choice of beverage, even when you are within your hours of eating.

ALCOHOL IS DEHYDRATING: Drinking alcohol dehydrates your body. Oddly enough, most of the time, a hangover is due, at least in part to dehydration. Therefore, if you are fasting and already struggling to keep yourself hydrated, it may not be a good idea to add insult to injury by drinking.

Alcohol Blocks Fat Breakdown: Alcohol is known to completely block the breakdown of fat. In one study the total of 19 adults were given an alcohol-rich. Even after five hours, the meal caused significantly reduced levels of fat breakdown. The control group were adults who consumed a meal that was rich in protein, fat, and carbs. So, basically, if you are putting all this work in to get healthier, and you drink, your full potential is impeded. All that hard work for the day is blunted and there is nothing you can do about it.

Alcohol may prevent cellular repair: While you are fasting, your body does its best to ramp up cellular repair. This process includes autophagy, which is extremely important for Intermittent Fasting to work. Autophagy is a process where old, damaged, or otherwise incompetint proteins are removed from cells. This makes room for the generation of new, healthier cells. This process is theorized to reduce the risk of cancer, promote anti-aging effects, and increase a human's lifespan.

The problem with alcohol, is that in recent studies performed on animals, indicate that high alcohol intake may inhibit autophagy. This is especially true for the in liver and fat tissue. While there are no studies completed yet on humans, regarding this theory, the possibility should be enough to convince people not to fast and drink heavily.

GRANTED, this is not to force people back into the times of prohibition. If you enjoy a drink or two during your non-fasting period, that is fine. It is just unwise to drink heavily. Once you are no longer fasting, if you choose to get off the fast at some point, you are more than welcome to do what you want. However, you do not want to forget that you will be a lighter individual, who has not drank in a while. Be warned that you might feel a buzz much sooner than what you're used to.

HOW TO OPTIMIZE INTERMITTENT FASTING AS A SENIOR

There are many benefits that are associated with Intermittent Fasting. To reach those benefits, though many people believe suffering is necessary. Thankfully, that is not the case. When you are Intermittently Fasting, there are sure to be some times of discomfort but that is it. There are plenty of hacks that help people of all ages optimize their Intermittent Fasting experience. Here are the hacks that have worked the best for individuals.

Drink Lots of Water

WHILE YOU ARE on your Intermittent Fasting journey, water will become your new best friend. It will help fill you up, keep you feeling good and help you focus. Everyone needs water but when you are

Intermittently Fasting, it is even more essential. For seniors, keeping a steady stream of water flowing through your body is good for helping your kidneys flush out the toxins that your fasting is pulling out of your stored fats. Plus, water helps to keep you vitalized and energetic. Drinking a lot of water will also keep the discomfort of fasting at bay.

Change Your Mindset

OUR MINDSET and the way we view a situation makes a big difference in how we feel about a situation. Think about it this way, if you are excited to go somewhere and the day finally comes, there is nothing that is going to make you have a bad day, as long as you get to go.

NOW, imagine you do not like going somewhere but you are going for your friend or significant other, because they enjoy it. If you think you are going to have a bad time, it doesn't matter what happens, as long as you are roped into going, you are going to be miserable.

INTERMITTENT FASTING IS the same way. If you are excited about this new journey and find ways to make it engaging for you, then the small inconveniences will not bother you. However, if you convince yourself it is going to be torture, it will be.

HERE ARE a few common ways that people can change their mindset and find adventure in the new experience:

INSTEAD OF: I can't eat breakfast/lunch...

THINK:

I have extra time to do whatever else I want to do.

I am saving so much money by eating less.

INSTEAD OF: I have to eat healthier…

THINK:

I have an opportunity to try something new.

PUTTING a positive spin on the otherwise negative aspects of Intermittent Fasting helps you get through the times of temptation and doubt. Plus, if you are able to do this effectively, it will add more conviction to your lifestyle change which will make it an all-around better experience.

Choose Your Own Timeframe

Everyone is different. It doesn't matter whether you work three jobs or you are retired, we all have a schedule. We all have times of the day where we are better, worse, tired, focused, relaxed and stressed. The good thing about Intermittent fasting is that you are able to choose the timeframe that is optimal for you, either to eat or fast. Yes, it is a block of time. However, there are options. The time of day that you fast doesn't matter, so long as you stick to that specific block of time.

THEREFORE, this lifestyle change is a lot easier to accomplish if you choose the time for eating and fasting that are optimal for your lifetime and your comfort. While most people use nighttime as the first leg of their journey, you can use it as your last. Or, if you work nights (or you are otherwise up at night) you can eat then. That is the beauty of this diet; you have options. If you make it work around your schedule, it will be a lot easier to form a routine.

Get Plenty of Sleep

Sleep is super important. While you are trying Intermittent Fasting, you need to sleep. Your body cannot function without proper sleep. It is true that generally, seniors need less sleep but that does not mean you can go without sleeping regularly, every day. Not only will sleep help get you through at least a few hours of fasting it will also ensure you are able to function while you are awake.

Eat Healthy

EATING HEALTHY SHOULD BE A GIVE-IN. Yet, given the "eat whatever you want" mindset that is sensationalized through the Intermittent Fasting coverage. Of course, everyone wants to be able to eat whatever they want and never get fat. The fact is, if you eat less of anything, you are going to lose weight. The problem is, will you be healthy? No. If all you consume is processed carbs and sugar, you are not giving your body what it needs to survive. All the fasting in the world is not going to save you from an early grave...but you will be skinny.

ALTERNATIVELY, eating healthy while being on an Intermittent Fasting diet is a hack, because it makes you feel a lot better. Eating fresh fruits and vegetables, meat, and yes, some carbs, will help you feel great! Giving your body what it needs is a big step toward helping your body cope with the changes you are putting it through. The more supportive you can be of your body, the better.

Walk

WALKING or any other form of exercise is excellent for Intermittent Fasting. It helps you burn calories (and fat) much more effectively. Walking is great because for most, seniors included, walking is an exercise that is not going to hurt you. It is not as stressful as running or weightlifting.

IF WALKING IS TOO strenuous for you, though, any type of movement will make you feel better. Ask you doctor what exercises would be beneficial to you. Follow their instructions and do not overdo it. If you do this, there is a good chance you will feel much better and the fasting experience will be far less harrowing.

AS YOU CAN SEE, some of these directions are more necessary than ordinary hacks. (The one about drinking water, specifically!) Yet, that does not mean they are any less hacks. However, they are not cheats. There is no cheating about these hacks.

These directives are not going to inhibit the effects of your fast in any way. These hacks are specifically designed to help you be healthier and happier throughout your fasting process. That way, the participant has an easier transition from dieting to changing their lifestyle for the better.

MINDSET FOR INTERMITTENT FASTING AS A SENIOR

When Intermittent Fasting, especially as a senior, it is important to remember that you are doing this to help yourself. Whichever method of Intermittent Fasting you choose, however you decide to break down the eating and fasting, remember that this is to make yourself healthier.

THEREFORE, if you push yourself too hard, or you find that you are not happier or feel better, you should stop doing it. There is often a fine line between encouraging yourself to keep going and knowing when you have had enough.

KNOW YOUR GOALS

. . .

GOALS. With all the different health benefits that are being linked to Intermittent Fasting, it is important to know exactly what you want out of your fasting experience. If you have goals, specific to your new, improved, happier lifestyle, it is easier to keep focused. Having a goal, when it comes to Intermittent Fasting means having a plan. If you know what you want to do, whether it is be healthier, lose weight, or simply gain more energy, it is important to impart that to your doctor, so that they can help you choose the right Intermittent Fasting lifestyle for you.

WHEN TO KNOW if Its Endurance or Hinderance:

THERE ARE many different ways to tell whether your body is telling you to keep going, or to cut it out. Although, sometimes those messages can become unclear, especially if you are dedicated to your cause. Here are a few considerations to take if you are unsure whether your body needs you to stick it out, or whether you should back off.

Listen to Your Doctor

Most people do not want to hear that they need to listen to their doctor but for seniors, listening to the advice of your doctor is crucial. Before you even start, you need to discuss your options with your doctor. If you and your physician mutually decide on an Intermittent Fasting plan, ask your doctor what you should expect. Hopefully, they will be able to give you some insight about what is normal for such a transition and what is unacceptable.

Time

TIME IS an important factor when it comes to conviction. The amount of time something is uncomfortable without improvement tells you that you are doing something that your body is NOT happy with. In this case, you want to stop what you're doing immediately. However, if you change your diet drastically, your body is going to react. Sometimes, that reaction is not pleasant. Although, once you get into a routine, you will get better. You might be hungry from time to time but the sensation of hunger being anywhere near unbearable should not exist for very long. Basically, once you commit yourself to fasting and think about it positively instead of dwelling on it, you should feel a difference.

· · ·

However, if at any time you feel something is wrong, eat immediately and talk to a doctor as soon as possible. That way, you will have assurance that what you are doing is right for you, personally.

Listen to Your Body

Pay attention to your body. When you are dieting, after you get past the fear that you are going to starve, you will start to notice that your body is telling you what it wants.

Have you ever had a craving for something completely random; possibly something that you have only had once or twice in your entire life? While that is indeed random, this is your body's way of telling you that it is lacking something that food had in it.

Usually, if you are hungry, you will grab whatever is easy and convenient. After all, as long as the hunger subsides, there is no reason to think about it anymore.

. . .

YET, when you are dieting; whether it is fasting or another healthy diet method, you are paying more attention to your body than ever before. Of course, you want to feel better, have more energy and look slimmer. Through that hyper-focus, you will also start to notice that your body is telling you what it requires. Likely your body will start helping you get it what it needs.

Do Not Fall into the All or Nothing Trap

MANY PEOPLE, with Intermittent Fasting, dieting in general, or mostly anything else, adopt an all or nothing attitude when it comes to what they are willing to do. In the case of Intermittent Fasting, people often push themselves beyond their limitations. Before they know it, they are tired of the changes and this causes them to stop altogether, returning to their old ways.

When it comes to any kind of lifestyle change, you do not want to fall into this category but this is particularly true for Intermittent Fasting.

Be Aware of Signs of Eating Disorders:

It is uncommon for someone to aspire to having an eating disorder. (Unfortunately, there are some people who are that crazy.) However, having or developing an eating disorder does not make a person crazy. Sadly, it is a fairly common. According to the National Association of Anorexia Nervosa and Associated Disorders (ANAD), at least 30 million people of all ages and genders suffer from an eating disorder in the U.S. That is men, women, and even children. Body morphing is not a new topic to our society but the dangers are only compounding.

WHEN PEOPLE THINK of eating disorders, Anorexia and Bulimia usually come to mind. However, there are many more different types of eating disorders that very few people talk about. One in particular is Orthorexia and it can become a concern for people who get deeply involved with Intermittent Fasting or other health plans.

WHAT IS ORTHOREXIA?

Orthorexia is a mental illness (eating disorder) that starts out as a lifestyle change. Most people who develop this illness simply want to eat healthier. However, before long, the person becomes consumed by the quality, ingredients, and preparation of their meals. A common way that people showcase this illness is by avoiding artificial colors, flavors, preservatives, pesticides, genetically modified products, fat, sugar, and salt, as well as animal and dairy products. Basically, people who are afflicted with this illness are obsessed with organic, home-grown foods, even to their own peril.

THOSE WHO SUFFER with the disorder are obsessed with what to eat and how much of it to eat, to achieve optimal health.

"THE MAIN DIFFERENCE between Orthorexia and other eating disorders is this idea that these behaviors are not for weight-loss purposes, but rather due to a belief that they are health-promoting," said Rachel Goldman, Ph.D., a clinical psychologist who focuses on wellness and disordered eating.

IRONICALLY, some of the noticeable symptoms of Orthorexia are malnutrition and severe weight loss. Simply because people afflicted with this illness are searching for prime health, does not mean that they find it. Unfortunately, many people with this illness are plagued with serious medical complications, as well as an impaired social, school, or work life.

SOMETIMES, Orthorexia gets so bad that victims of the sickness refuse to let anyone else prepare their meals. They need to know where everything comes from and cannot think about anything else.

YET, even if you see their unhealthiness starting to show through, they don't see it. Much like other eating disorders, people with Orthorexia see themselves differently. They think they look healthy. They have convinced themselves that all of their research and their meticulous food preparation is helping them and everyone else is wrong.

PROTECTING **Yourself**

BEING aware of eating disorders is a step in the right direction to helping those afflicted and protecting yourself against slipping into a similar situation. Remember, the most alarming pitfall of Orthorexia is that the people who become afflicted are simply trying to do the right thing. They are trying to make themselves healthier. It isn't about being a model or appearance. It starts with a desire to be healthy. There is no get-slim fast tricks that make them sick. They are not taking supplements or doing something to their bodies that cause them to get sick. They just become obsessed with being healthy.

When it comes to Intermittent Fasting, there is

definitely a risk of falling into a similar frame of mind. After all, regardless of the support system you have, unless you have people who are also fasting with you, you are going at it alone. Everyone around you, everyone that you know, even if they support you, are eating completely different than you. Sometimes, this can cause people to feel isolated. If that isolation gets to be too much, you might think that you know better than everyone else. Fact and figments of your own mind start to fuse, causing you to lose touch with reality.

That is why it is so important to keep a healthy check on reality throughout your fasting and dieting process. It is slippery slopes like this that can take a normal, even positive action and turn it into something that completely destroys their life.

Fortunately, if a person keeps in regular contact with their doctor and listens to what they say, there is a much better chance that they will stay on the right path; a path that is both healthy for the body and the mind.

ALTERNATE TYPES OF
INTERMITTENT FASTING

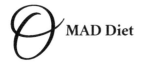MAD Diet

THE ONE MEAL A Day Diet, or, the much more
mysterious name, the OMAD diet, draws people in
with a simple premise: (Cue annoying announcer
voice:) To lose weight, feel better, and save money,
eat only one meal per day!

OH BOY.

TO MAKE IT MORE APPEALING, though, (because who
wants to just eat one meal per day) with the OMAD
diet, you can eat whatever you want! Choose wisely,

though, because as soon as that wears off you're going to starve until the next day's dinner time.

WHAT MAKES this work is that there is only so much food a person can eat in one sitting. (Please, do not take that as a challenge.) That is the only reason you "can eat whatever you want" and still manage to lose weight. Chalorically, it is a lot harder to eat an over abundance of food during one meal. Plus, if you are eating less (one meal) your body is going to start demanding less to function.

THE OMAD DIET is really just the overachievers Intermittent Fasting. Ultimately, there is good reason why people are not too keen on trying this form of dieting; it is super intense. While most of the Intermittent Fasting regimens use sleep as a way to lessen the amount of hunger a person feels, the OMAD diet forces people to get through sleeping and an entire day before having a bite to eat.

THE IDEOLOGY:

ACCORDING to OMAD enthusiasts and a few studies, claim that there are benefits to this diet.

- **Increased focus and productivity:** The increased focus and productivity that is experienced through this diet is created from two combined forces. The first, is that the longer you fast, the more Noradrenaline your body is producing. This keeps you sharp and focused. Back in the days of cavemen and cavewomen, this alertness made it possible for you to continue to hunt, even when you were running low on food. It helped you get a meal, instead of becoming a meal. Now, it helps you get through the day without passing out. The second, is the inability to succumb to a food coma. The afternoon slump is supposedly non existent, because there is no food to slow you down.

- **Weight Loss:** This is kind of a given. Again, people can only eat so much at one time. Even if they have not eaten all day, there is still only so much room for food in a person's stomach. Thus, it is difficult to over-indulge if you are only eating one meal a day. This is ultimately what allows dieters to be able to eat "whatever they want" during their one meal and still lose weight. Ultimately, it is forcing yourself to not overeat, both mentally and physically.

Yet, that still doesn't mean that eating whatever you want is a healthy choice.

- **Freeing You From Common Diet Hangups:** This is more of a convenience than an actual benefit, but it is still not a bad thing. Since you are only eating one meal per day while participating in the OMAD diet, you don't have to focus on counting calories. Therefore, you can eat like a king and still lose weight but only if you do it once per day.

- **Successful Navigation of this Diet Helps Willpower and Discipline:** If a person can successfully navigate the OMAD diet for an extended period of time, you will take away a powerful gift of willpower and discipline that is sure to help you with your weight loss goals. Ultimately, the secret to breaking the cycle of indulgence is the lack of willpower. If you can resist the temptation to eat, especially when your body is telling you how hungry you are, you will be able to resist the temptation after you have stopped dieting. As long as you do not give in to the desire to eat everything to make up for the time you ate hardly anything, you should be able to maintain that willpower with relative ease.

THE PROBLEM with these studies is that they are not specific to the OMAD diet. These studies all cite "Intermittent Fasting" as the beneficiary diet model, not specifically the OMAD diet. The second issue is directly related to the first; there is not enough information on the OMAD diet to specifically say that putting yourself through this torture is worth it.

ISSUES WITH THE **OMAD** DIET:

THIS DIET SEEMS EXTREME. Seniors, as well as people of all ages should be cautious when trying this heavy-duty fasting diet. While it might be a good way to lose weight, it can be detrimental to your health, depending on the types of medical conditions the participant is diagnosed with. Even if the benefits help your blood pressure and circulatory system, a person must be healthy enough to keep fasting, if nothing else, to get those benefits.

ABOVE, the benefits of the OMAD Diet were laid out. Now, here are the issues with the diet:

Eating Whatever You Want Might Not Be the Best Idea:

For an adult who has struggled with their weight, the idea of being able to eat whatever you want is a freeing experience. The idea that you will still lose weight, even if you eat everything in sight, so long as you only do it once a day...That might be enough of an incentive to actually complete a few days worth of such an extreme diet. BUT for anyone who is trying to lose weight, their goal should also (more importantly) be to get healthy. Eating junk food for the entirety of your meal might still allow you to lose weight but it will not make you healthy.

A PERSON who is engaging in this diet, especially a senior, has much more at stake than a weight issue. Unhealthy eating habits could create or severely worsen the conditions you already have; even if you are only eating one meal per day.

ADDITIONALLY, the medical benefits that are associated with Intermittent Fasting are non-existent if you do not provide your body with anything useful to work with. If you give your body nothing but junk, you might lose weight but you will still feel terrible. At that point, you are simply filling a void that happens to get smaller. You won't starve but you won't feel good either. You might just waste away.

. . .

THE APPEAL FOR SENIORS:

DO NOT MISCONSTRUE, this could work out great for seniors, who are able to both eat balanced diets, eat a fair amount of food at once, and get the right caloric intake. However, depending on how your body reacts to food, that could be a difficult task. With this in mind, there could be an appeal to this diet for seniors that is not such a good thing. As people get older, they sometimes lose the ability to taste food as purely as they once could. Thus, food becomes less appetizing. For some, eating could even become a chore.

IF THIS HAPPENS, seniors might revel in the idea of only having to eat once per day. The problem with this is when people are unwilling to eat, their intake for when they do eat is severely limited. Many seniors are not physically capable of consuming the right amount of calories for this diet to be healthy for them.

ALTERNATE-DAY FASTING

THE PERSON who is credited with this type of Intermittent Fasting is Krista Varady, PhD, a nutrition professor at the University of Illinois. This is an interesting alternative to other methods, as it encourages dietors to fast every other day. Unlike other methods that demand a lot of calories per day, during a shorter time period. This fasting method enables people to eat only twenty-five percent of their normal calorie needs, which is only about 500 calories, on fasting days. However on feasting days, or non-fasting days, people are encouraged to eat as they normally would. (Although, enacting a balanced diet is definitely a good idea for prolonged health.

In addition to Dr. Varaday, another popular influencer that is taking over the YouTube scene on this subject is Rachel Sharp.

According to these and other Alternate-Day Fasting gurus, this is a popular approach for weight loss.

THE IDEOLOGY:

THIS IS a diet that has gotten a lot of attention and even specific studies, but it still remains fairly elusive. Nevertheless, the benefits that this alleges makes it extremely appealing, primarally to people who are obese.

- **Weight Loss:** Yes, all Intermittent Fasting diets are about losing weight. However, this specific type of Intermittent Fasting is especially important because there is a study that singles this method out specifically. There was a small study published in *Nutrition Journal* by Dr. Varady and colleagues way back in 2010. The study found alternate day fasting was conclusively effective in helping obese adults in particular lose weight. Throughout the study, it was found that most severe hunger side-effects became manageable within two weeks. This is about the same ten-day period that many of the other Intermittent Fasting methods give for side effects to subside. After about a month, the participants started to feel more satisfied with their overall experience. This study lasted eight-weeks and the most common issue was that participants claimed they never really felt "full".

- **Lower Cholesterol Levels:** Cholesterol is a serious issue for seniors, particularly if they are overweight. Therefore, to have a diet within the Intermittent Fasting spectrum that lowers cholesterol is a major win. Plus, these levels were lowered while still maintaining a fairly "normal" diet for the participants. That means that people are still able to enjoy their favorite foods, just not as often.

- **Reduced Levels of a Biological Marker:** This biological marker is associated with inflammation and age-associated disease. What this means, is Alternate -Day Fasting opens the door to further research about lowering inflammation and adding to longevity, even in people who are considered obese. If this proves to be a long-term diet that people who are obese can stick to, this could end up being a life-saving medical gem that we are just mining. The potential in this and other health benefits from this method of Intermittent Fasting is very exciting to the nutrition community.

- **Increased Ketone Bodies:** These ketone bodies are not only responsible for garnering energy from the body, produced by burning fat, they are also theorized to be essential to a person's overall health. What is interesting about the production of ketone bodies while a person is on the Alternate-Day Fasting diet, is that the rate of production continues even on non-fasting days. This means that the process of burning fat and promoting overall health is diligently working throughout every day of the diet.

ISSUES WITH THE ALTERNATE-DAY FASTING:

ALTERNATE-DAY FASTING IS OFTEN at the root of all studies, both good and bad, when it comes to Intermittent Fasting. Despite this there is still extremely limited information about the effects, both good and bad of alternative fasting or other Intermittent Fasting methods. Nevertheless, here are the known issues with Alternate-Day Fasting:

RESEARCH IS LIMITED

"STRICT ADF IS one of the most extreme diet interventions, and it has not been sufficiently investigated within randomized controlled trials," said Frank Madeo, a professor of the Institute of Molecular Biosciences at Karl-Franzens University of Graz in Austria. This is coming nine years after the initial study conducted by ADF cheerleader, Dr. Varaday. This statement was a precursor to Dr.

Madeo's own study, published in the Cell Press in August 2019.

THE GOOD NEWS is that all of Dr. Varaday's benefits were substantiated by Dr. Madeo's trial. Plus, the new study was able to bring some previously-known benefits into clearer focus. According to the study, here are the positive results:

- *"They had continuous upregulation of ketone bodies, even on non-fasting days. This has been shown to promote health in various contexts."* While there is nothing new here, it is still nine years later and the findings concur the first study, completed in 2010.
- *"They had reduced levels of sICAM-1, a marker linked to age-associated disease and inflammation."* This is a little more in-depth than the original study, naming the biological marker that is responsible for age-related disease and inflammation. Still, however, the information that is revealed only adds to the study's predecessor's findings.
- *"They had lowered levels of triiodothyronine without impaired thyroid gland function. Previously, lowered levels of this hormone have*

been linked to longevity in humans." This is a newer finding altogether, that may have been suspected but not confirmed.

- *"They had lowered levels of cholesterol."* This was another finding that was consistent with the study conducted in 2010.
- *"They had a reduction of lipotoxic android trunk fat mass."* This is a very long and scientific way of saying belly fat. All this means is that the people who participated in the study had a reduction of belly fat. In other words, they lost weight. This too was a finding that was first introduced by the original, widespread study.

HOWEVER, even with all these benefits, the issue remained for Dr. Madeo that he could not conclusively support this diet. Dr. Madeo believes that there is still much more research to be done. While that is not inherently a bad thing, it is discouraging for people who are hopeful that trying this diet will work for them.

This Encourages Binge Eating

The idea that the people in the study could never feel the sensation of being full is scary. People do not like to not feel full and for someone who is obease, the inability to feel full could lead to some extremely bad habits. Sure, if they are still on the diet, they are eating less but if they do not eat the right foods, they could be at major risk for other developing health issues.

ERRATIC "ANYTHING GOES" hunger-centered fasting.

A good rule, generally, is that erratic is not a good description when it comes to anything medical or health-related. *Erratic* is not a good description to be placed in front of mental health, physical health, emotional health, or any other health one can come up with. The connotation that erratic holds does not offer much confidence in any capacity. Yet, it is considered a method of Intermittent Fasting.

THE IDEOLOGY:

THE IDEOLOGY that guides this interesting form of Intermittent Fasting is listening to your body. While that is not bad advice, it does not evoke much stability. After all, this method is appropriately named. This method is centered around eating when you are hungry and fasting when you are not hungry. This method helps the person using it break the conventions of mealtime. For instance, you are supposed to eat when you are hungry, instead of eating because it is luchtime, or dinnertime, or breakfast time. Much like the rest of the Intermittent Fasting methods, this one does promote a healthy diet. Plus, it is extremely important for a person to listen to a medical professional's advice when adhering to this diet, because at least that will add some structure.

HERE ARE the benefits of Erratic Fasting:

- **You Are Not Eating Unnecessarily:**
  Freeing yourself from the conformity of a meal "time" is helpful on your weight loss journey. If you are not hungry at a specific time, that means your body is not in need of anything. When you are hungry, you are answering your body's call. This could certainly be beneficial. Additionally, since you are not eating as a result of conformity, you are freeing yourself from social norms and thus, helping yourself to become more social and less reliant on food as a buffer. Even if you go out with friends, you are voluntarily removing a lifejacket for the sea of conversation that will exist. This could result in more confidence and self-assurance.
- **You are Practicing Listening to Your**

Body: Listening to your body is what this Intermittent Fasting method is all about. This method gives you the chance to learn what your body truly wants. This diet gives you free-range to learn about yourself. Ultimately, most people do this to be healthier but that only works if you are able to successfully tune into your body's needs, instead of caving to every whim and want your consciousness has.

- **It gives You an Opportunity to Follow Your Own Path:** Following your own path is extremely important and for some people, that is the only way to live. That is why, for some people, this "erratic" fasting method works because it allows people to make their own decisions. Yet, it still has some semblance of guidelines to help the person make a healthier, more personalized choice about their own consumption habits.

ISSUES WITH ERRATIC FASTING:

There are problems with Erratic Fasting, as you could imagine. Most of those issues come from the diet's free-spirited nature. That does not mean that it doesn't work. It simply means the lack of guide-lines makes it extremely difficult to control.

There is No Rhyme or Reason to the Diet:

Essentially, the diet is a free-for-all. The whole point of the diet is to eat when you're hungry. While it is a great lesson in non-conformity, it is not an overly-effective diet. Specifically, the reason is that the people on this diet do not know how to eat (or refuse to eat correctly). That is why they feel the need to go on a diet. If people could control them-selves, they would be able to manage their weight and health without 'dieting'. Therefore, giving people who need clear direction to be healthier an abstract, highly personalized direction and calling it a diet is not conducive to their health. People want to go down the path of least resistance and the brain can convince people of a lot. If they think they are dieting, when really, they are just eating whenever they want, that is not helping them.

There are No Significant Studies:

The reason there are no significant studies, specifically targeting Erratic Fasting is because it is over-personalized. There is no real way to accu-rately judge what a group of people are doing and if their results correlate to the diet, because everyone is different. There is no direction that everyone has to follow. People get hungry at different times of the day. So, short of a log, created by the participant, there is little else that researchers would even have to go on for data collection.

Ultimately, this form of 'dieting' should be reserved for people who are already in control of their weight. While there is merit in only eating when you are hungry, not just because it is conventionally time for a meal, it is hard to believe that people without immense self-control can tell the difference between needing to eat and wanting to eat. Due to this, there are a lot of pitfalls that could actually make this diet dangerous. So, while it is not outrightly risky, as a senior, it is advised to be very careful if you try this method.

7 MISTAKES PEOPLE MAKE AND HOW TO AVOID THEM

*F*asting is hard. Even when it is working and you are having success from the experience, it is difficult. Again, Intermittent Fasting is a lifestyle change. It takes patience, understanding, time, and even a few adjustments along the way to make it work. This goes for anyone who is starting Intermittent Fasting. Here are 7 Mistakes that people make when they first start out with their intermittent fasting and how to avoid those mistakes:

#1: Too Much Too Fast:

REGARDLESS OF WHETHER your goals are weight loss, healthier living, building muscle mass, or something else entirely, dieting is a marathon, not a race. You have to work really hard to achieve your goal. No one is going to wake up one morning and be in stellar shape, having met all their goals after one day of dieting. It takes months, sometimes years to achieve the goals people set for themselves. Even though Intermittent Fasting can get you results, this is not a get healthy quick scheme. Much like the other diets that genuinely work for people, you have to commit to it.

THEREFORE, with the idea of having a long-term commitment in mind, it makes sense that you do not want to jump in with both feet. You cannot go from zero to sixty on this and expect for it to be a pleasant experience. Even though your body wants to be healthy, it is stuck in a rut of being unhealthy. You have habits that you need to break and your body is accustomed to those habits. That is why the first mistake that people make, on day one, is going from eating frequently to fasting.

WHILE YOU LIKELY WILL NOT HAVE ANY life-threatening effects, you are more likely to stop and return to your old ways, because nothing changed. Say you make it a week-that was one of the worst weeks of your life, but since your mindset didn't change, your body continued to yearn for more food. So, when you say the hunger and aggravation aren't worth the results, you will default back to your old ways.

AVOIDING THIS MISTAKE:

A good way to avoid this mistake is to ease into it. You do not have to go from eating every four hours to only eating for one third of the day. Instead, work your way up to it. Build mini-milestones so you can see yourself progressing without feeling like you're starving yourself. Try to go for six hours at a time without eating. Then, go eight, ten, and twelve hours without eating. Eventually, work your way up to fasting for the full sixteen hours. If you do it this way, your transition will be a lot smoother than if you just cut off your body's sustenance in a day.

#2: Not Drinking Enough Water

This portion was covered briefly earlier; water is more important than food. Water makes up sixty percent of the human body's composition. Our brain, heart, lungs, and even our bones are made up of a solid percentage of water. Water is important because each and every cell in our body is dependant on it. Food, while essential, is not even part of this list. We, in fact, are not what we eat; at least, not in this sense. Water is ultimately what makes us feel better or worse, depending on our level of hydration.

THUS, a large portion of success while fasting is drinking the right amount of water, to help make up for the absence of food. When our body starts working harder, breaking into our reserve of stored energy: body fat, (not muscle) it needs more water to help it function.

WATER IS what helps our bodies feel better, look younger, and work harder. Any diet or health professional will stress the importance of water. While hunger does not make you lose energy, the symptoms that are generally associated with starvation are actually due to dehydration. It does not take a long time for a person to become dehydrated. When that happens, people feel weak, sick, tired, and develop aches and pains.

WHILE THIS COULD BE CONSIDERED a crude example, water for humans (and most living creatures) is like oil for a car. It lubricates everything and ensures that parts of the body, from ligiements to organs, do not get stuck due to being dried out. Water replenishes our vitalization and helps us to get through everything. People can live for a long time without food. People cannot generally live more than a week without water. (Most people will not be able to make it more than three or four days. The reasoning is that more than half of our body's composition is cut off, without water.

OF COURSE, people are not going to intentionally dehydrate themselves. Yet, it is surprisingly easy to not get enough water, especially while fasting.

Avoiding this Mistake:

In order to avoid this mistake, because this is one you really do not want to make, drink the right amount of water. A good goal is to drink four or five liters per day, to ensure you are getting the right amount of water while you are fasting. Additionally, it is important to get used to drinking a good amount of water daily, before starting your fast. That way, the change is one less thing you need to get used to during your fast. Plus, it might help you make the transition easier.

*PRO TIP: Drinking sparkling water will not break your fast but it will help you to feel full quicker.

#3: Becoming Consumed with Fasting:

Fasting is a big change. It is a lifestyle change. If you do it correctly, chances are you will be able to continue it long-term. After all, once you get over the hungry hump (of about a month) and your body adjusts, there is little reason to stop doing what works. Since this is not a short-term slim-down, Intermittent Fasting can become a permanent routine, if you want.

WITH THIS IN MIND, though, it is important that you do not allow fasting to rule your life. Think about it, when you eat breakfast, lunch, and dinner now, do you overthink it? No. You work around whatever comes up in your life.

THE GOOD THING about intermittent fasting is that it is not a diet that is set in stone. It can be manipulated and worked around. You want to find a way that Intermittent Fasting works with your lifestyle. You cannot be a slave to it, or you will end up resenting it. Instead, if you have to rearrange your fasting hours, or if you accidentally break a fast, it is okay. Remember, there is always tomorrow and if your fasting plan does not go as planned one day, it does not erase all the hard work you put in up to that point. You can always get back on track.

Avoiding this Mistake:

Do not treat fasting as though you are going to get flogged if you cheat or mess up. Remember, you are doing this to better your own life, not serve a new master. You want to feel good and part of that is being flexible enough with your fasting to make it work for you. Do not cancel plans with friends and family, or avoid doing something you enjoy, simply because of your fast. The whole point of feeling better is to be able to enjoy life more, not less. There is always a way around it, or a new day to start over. Your happiness is not exclusive to your weight loss. It is merely a portion of a well-rounded lifestyle.

#4: Completely Turning Your World Upside Down:

FASTING, by itself, is difficult. Change is difficult. However, even though we know this, sometimes, when we finally decide what our plan of action is going to be, we go overboard with it. Instead of pacing themselves, they dive headfirst into an entirely different lifestyle. While this is generally a good thing for you, it is still not a good idea to flip the script on your entire life. After all, you are used to feeling a certain way and doing certain things. If you wake up one day and do everything different, your body is going to revolt. When this happens, it is extremely possible that you are going to feel much worse before you feel even the slightest bit better.

. . .

THERE ARE many different reasons why someone would want to try Intermittent Fasting. The health benefits are one reason, weight loss is another reason, and some people do it to gain muscle. Therefore, they work out. However, when you are eating less, working out more, and completely changing your diet, you are putting your body into overload. While all of these things might be good for your body, working out is stressful on your body. Trying to adhere to a new food regimen is stressful on your body. On top of that, you cannot stop your life, so that you can get used to being on a new food regimen. You need to be able to make it work for your lifestyle.

AVOIDING THIS MISTAKE:

DO NOT GET THIS WRONG, it is important to have a healthy diet while you are Intermittently Fasting. This is not a quick fix. It is a way to train your body to only ask for what it needs. However, getting in over your head and changing too many things at once will only set you up for failure. This is why it is important to implement big changes slowly. Eat a healthy diet but take advantage of the times or days that you are able to eat. Make sure you hit the calorie count each time frame you are supposed to eat and if your body wants something specific, let yourself enjoy it. The cool thing about Intermittent Fasting is that you do not have to worry so much about what you eat. As long as you are incorporating a balanced diet into your eating habits, you are good to go. Get used to fasting before intensifying your workout. Focus on how your body feels before you add on any more changes.

#5: Maintaining the Lifestyle of the Couch Potato

Overeating leads to a sluggish disposition. Therefore, we become couch potatoes. We do not do much more than sit and eat. The television is a large part of our daily entertainment. While there is nothing wrong with enjoying a show, the couch should not be our preferred center for enjoyment.

THIS IS ESPECIALLY true when you start to have more energy. You have to do something or you are going to get bored very easily. When you get bored, you get frustrated. Energy has to do something and if it is not burnt off in a productive manner, it festers into something unpleasant.

.   .   .

Plus, whether you are dieting or not, you are not doing your body any favors by not doing anything.

Avoiding this Mistake:

The best way to avoid this mistake is to enjoy life! This can be a fun and creative way to make your new, healthy lifestyle work for you. If you have never been an active person, start small and work your way up. Go for a walk, try a workout class, or take part in a sport. You don't have to break any records or commit to anything major. Even dancing in your living room is better than sitting on the couch all day. Once you get yourself moving, you will be happy with the way you feel and what you are able to accomplish.

In fact, making yourself get up and go will likely give you more energy. If you find ways to keep yourself busy, you will also have less time to overthink either your hunger or your fasting. Filling your days with adventure and trying new things will help you feel better quicker and see positive results sooner.

#6: Trying to Fast Alone

Even if you do not have anyone down in the trenches, actually fasting alongside of you, it is still important to take advantage of the support of friends and family. You do not want to try to take this journey alone. It is hard enough, with love, support, and encouragement.

HOWEVER, when people try to change their lifestyle, even for the better, there is a sense of embarrassment that can come along with it. Common thoughts that people have are: *What if I fail? I'd rather nobody knows until I start seeing results. I don't want to have to answer to anyone else when I go out.*

LET'S look at them one by one:

WHAT IF I FAIL?

THE GOOD NEWS about this is the only way to fail is by giving up. You are trying to better your life and your health. There is nothing wrong with that. If you stumble, you are going to want support to get back up and try again tomorrow.

YOU CAN BE your most difficult and even hurtful critic. When you are in doubt, it is nice to have someone there, standing by your side, ready to pick you up and bring you back to reality. Knowing that

you are not alone is key. Even if they are not participating in the diet with you, simply having someone
to talk to and an encouraging word does a lot to help
pull you out of your times of doubt.

I'D RATHER nobody knows until I start seeing results.

SPEAKING as someone who has struggled with my
weight in the past, this is completely understandable.
Getting compliments for what you have done is
much better than being questioned about what you
are doing. The trial and error of some diets can
make people who are close to you react more nega-
tively than supportive. They can make you feel like
you aren't trying or that if the diet doesn't work for
you, you have somehow failed *them.*

MOST OF THE TIME, hopefully, their comments come
from a place of concern, instead of blatantly aiming
to be hurtful. Yet, their intention matters little when
you feel like you are being called out. After all, you
obviously wished the diet worked way more than
they could ever know. So, their portrayal of disap-
pointment is like rubbing salt in a wound; a big,
glaringly obvious, wound.

. . .

HOWEVER, if someone reacts that way, or has reacted that way in the past, take it as a cue that you should not tell them about your weight loss journeys. That doesn't mean, however, that you should keep it a secret. If you do not have anyone in your circle of friends who can manage to be supportive, go to or get involved in a support group. The people who are in such a support group, whether it is online or in-person, is likely looking for the same type of encouragement that you are. Therefore, they will be understanding and who knows, you might even meet some new friends!

I DON'T WANT to have to answer to anyone else when I go out.

AGAIN, it is nice to think that when loved ones comment on certain areas of your personal life, especially in relation to losing weight, that they are speaking from a place of concern. It is possible that they have your best interest at heart. Yet, that does not make their glaring eyes and disappointed expression any easier to stand when they question you about being on a diet.

EVEN AFTER THIS HAPPENS ONCE, it is generally

enough to embarrass you enough that you never want to be put in that position again. Unfortunately, if you know that person you likely will not be able to get away from them that easily.

IF YOU REFRAIN from discussing your dieting and they still make comments that make you feel uncomfortable, talk to them. Explain how you are feeling and if they truly care, they will make adjustments. If they don't then you probably do not need them in your life. After all, any period of growth demands change, both inwardly and outwardly. While you shouldn't go looking to axe friendships and relationships, sometimes it is necessary. After all, you are changing your entire lifestyle.

Avoiding this Mistake:

Fasting alone doesn't work. Therefore, it is important to find a supporter (or a group of supporters) that can talk to you freely and openly. You don't want them to placate you but you do want them to be willing to encourage you outwardly. Whether this comes from a friend or relationship you already have or from joining a support group, it is important that you do not try to try Intermittent Fasting alone.

#7: Accidentally Breaking Your Fast

It can be difficult to fast. Fasting, with the explicit purpose of denying your body food so that it uses up stored energy (fat) goes against our natural instinct. It is taking one of the main pillars of our basic needs and using it against ourselves. Fasting takes willpower and endurance, as well as a conscious effort to avoid food (and still live a normal life.) That is not an easy thing to do.

EVEN THOUGH THE concept of fasting sounds simple: Don't eat, there is a lot of small details that make this diet harder than most. One of the hardest issues is breaking your fast without even realizing you have done so.

SINCE THIS DIET is based specifically on how long you don't eat, opposed to watching what you do eat, issues are sure to arise. However, when you take the idea of not eating and couple it with the need to consume water (and select other beverages) the once cut and dry directive gets murky. For instance, people hear the word "fast" and they think *don't eat.* Great. That's perfect.

WELL, what about drinking?

. . .

YOU HAVE to drink water and to save yourself from a major caffeine headache, you are able to drink coffee and tea. The problem is that people put things in their water, coffee, and tea that break their fast. Some of the obvious additions to water, coffee, and tea is lemon, milk, and sugar...Oh, and apparently, some people put butter in their coffee. From a coffee drinker who actually likes the taste of coffee (I'm an alien, I know) that comes across as extremely strange.

HOWEVER, the point is that many people hear they are supposed to or are allowed to drink certain liquids and automatically add whatever they normally would to those liquids. That is breaking the fast.

NOW, is breaking a fast the end of the world? No. It will lessen the effects of the fast for the day, but it will not completely negate all your hard work.

STILL, if you do this every day, you are still working really hard for diluted results.

Avoiding this Mistake:

This mistake can be remedied by thinking before you consume anything. Plain water, you're good to go. Black coffee, great! Plain tea? Perfect. If you go to do anything else, make sure you run it through a quick Google search to make sure whatever you want to do is not adding any calories to your intake.

AFTER ALL, it is the calories that break a fast.

HOW EXERCISE AIDS
INTERMITTENT FASTING

*E*xercise is the key to unlocking the true potential of Intermittent Fasting. This chapter reiterates the importance of exercise. This not only a hack, though. While it will definitely make you feel better, it is not the only way that exercise aids the Intermittent Fasting process.

THE ODD THING is that there are many different opinions about exercising while fasting. However, the opinions that lean toward negativity are usually based heavily on performance. More often for seniors, though, they want to know whether exercising is a good thing to do while participating in Intermittent Fasting.

· · ·

BENEFITS

EVERYONE IS TOLD NOT to work out on an empty stomach. However, as it turns out, there are a lot of advantages to working out this way. While the idea is not the most renowned, (after all, working out *and* not having food in your system sounds lethal!) Fortunately, it is not. In fact, many people who work out during Intermittent Fasting (while fasting) have found a plethora of benefits.

Improved Insulin Sensitivity

Intermittent Fasting is proven to increase your insulin sensitivity. Insulin is what helps your cells receive the glucose from your food. When Your insulin sensitivity is low, your body reacts in a negative manner. Here are some of the most common symptoms of insulin sensitivity:

- Fatigue
- Weight Gain
- Patches of dark skin
- Elevated fasting blood sugar
- Acne
- Sugar and carb cravings
- Feeling angry whenever you are hungry or "hangry"
- Scalp hair loss in women

- Skin tags
- High blood pressure
- Fluid retention
- Trouble concentrating

SINCE SOCIETY HAS CONVINCED us that there are so many different reasons for all of these symptoms, people do not know there is even a problem. Some people even believe that a lot of these symptoms, like being hangry, is a product of their personality. Therefore, they learn to deal with it instead of unlocking their full potential of energy.

THE GOOD NEWS IS, Intermittent Fasting helps increase the resistance a person's body has to Insulin Sensitivity. As a result, many of these side effects will go away. That could mean a host of physical and internal changes that will make you happier with yourself and feel better.

Recovery from Endurance Exercise

It is theorized that working out, while in a fasting state, actually improves post-workout recovery. Through endurance-heavy exercise, participants were able to recover quicker, maintain muscle mass, lower fat mass, and maintain their level of performance. This is an interesting theory and another idea that completely turns what we thought we knew about fitness on its head.

Improved Recovery from Weight Training

A 2009 study found that participants who lifted weights in a fasted state enjoyed a greater "intramyocellular anabolic response" to the post-workout meal. The levels of p70s6 kinase doubled. (p70s6 is a muscle protein synthesis signaling mechanism which basically indicates muscle growth.)

Improved Glycogen Repletion and Retention

Glycogen is synthesized from glucose at times where blood glucose levels are high. This is in preparation for when glucose levels are low, at which time, Glycogen serves as a backup source of glucose to give muscles the power they need to perform. Of course, when you are fasting, eventually, even the Glycogen is gone and the body must resort to using the stored fat as an energy source.

WHEN THE STORED fat becomes the source of energy for the body, the performance of the person may be less than stellar. However, it is theorized that Glycogen is replaced and able to be used longer after fasting. After all, our body is always adapting. If we put our bodies in a situation where it constantly needs more Glycogen, it will adapt. It will start to pack away more Glycogen, so that we will be more capable of working at our best potential at all times.

. . .

THE IDEA behind this is that if your body is able to perform while it is at a high level of fat burning for energy, your body will only perform better when it has fuel. Yet, there are others who believe that this type of exercise is better because there is nothing slowing down your body.

(THIS IS the same idea as those who believe the afternoon idus is cured by not eating lunch.) Basically, if there is no food in your system to slow you down, you will continue to perform at your peak.

STILL, many people maintain that fasted exercise does not need to be difficult. Training is supposed to prepare you for your competition. It is not always supposed to break you. To add credence to that, our own body shows us this is true by the benefits it provides us.

MANY OF THE known benefits of fasted exercise are achieved at the pace of a light, aerobic workout, in a state of glycogen depletion. This could be the result of a 30-minute walk or hike, a simple swim, or even yoga.

. . .

OF COURSE, many seniors who are thinking of partaking in Intermittent Fasting are not worried about performance or growing their muscles. Yet, this information is still important, because it allows seniors to strive for greatness. The stronger you make yourselves, the easier it is for your body to overcome your ailments. The older people get, the more they need help keeping their muscles working properly. If you are already working towards the goal of maintaining your strength, any deterioration is going to be slowed significantly.

SOMETIMES, you do not know how powerful you can be, until you set your mind to it.

KETO AND INTERMITTENT FASTING

*O*riginally, the Keto Diet (also known as the Ketogenic Diet) was first a way to help children suffering from epilepsy.The classic keto diet a very low-carb, moderate-protein, and high-fat diet. It typically contains 75% fat, 20% protein and only 5% carbs. The name ketogenic or keto comes from the idea that the diet produces ketones in the body. Research shows that higher ketone levels result in better seizure control. The only reason this diet is primarily recommended for children is because adults find it too difficult.

IN MOST CASES, our bodies use carbohydrates for energy. Carbs primarily comes from bread and pasta but they are found in other foods as well. The keto diet forces the body to switch from using carbs for entergy, to using fats for energy. Even though it is not the 'normal' source of energy, our bodies are able to adapt well to utilizing ketones and fats in lieu of carbs.

SHOULD you combine the keto diet and Intermittent Fasting? That depends on your goals and your health. There is no doubt that the goals of both dieting methods are interchangable. Thus, it makes sense that putting them together will make the overall process more successful. Here are some benefits of combining the keto diet and Intermittent Fasting:

May Smooth Your Path to Ketosis

Combining the keto and Intermittent Fasting method of your choice could help your body reach ketosis quicker and easier than either diet by itself. The reason for this is that when a person is fasting, their body maintains its energy balance by switching its fuel source from carbs to fats. People on the keto diet have the same goal; giving your body more fat than carbs for a prolonged period of time.

THIS TOO GOES BACK to the time of the caveman, when people were either the hunter or the hunted. There was no in-between, so they needed to have an alternative source of energy to continue moving and thinking, when food was scarce. That is why sustinece is not our body's exclusive energy producer.

THIS IS a possible option for people who struggle to reach ketosis while on a keto or Intermittent Fasting diet. Combining the two can help skyrocket your body into ketosis and effectively pave your path to weight loss and health

May Lead to More Fat Loss

IT DOES MAKE SENSE, that the more diets you are on, the more fat is lost in a given time. Yet, unlike many different diets, with Intermittent Fasting and the keto diet, it is possible to not only survive, but thrive while practicing both at the same time. Since this leads to more fat loss, this could also be a great motivator for the person who needs to see results to be encouraged.

ADDITIONALLY, there was a study that found Intermittent Fasting could help protect mice from diet-induced metabolic abnormalities. Basically, the study found that Intermittent Fasting was able to minimize the negative effects the low-calorie diet was having on the subject's metabolism. The keto diet helped the mice lose weight but the Intermittent fasting (specifically alternate-day fasting) allowed enough time for their bodies to compensate for the decreased body weight reduced amount of food. Therefore, the two diets worked together to create an epic health and weight loss promoting regimine.

Side Effects

Keep in mind that both of these diets on their own can be a major change and a complete shock to your system. Additionally, it is not necessary to do both the keto diet *and* Intermittent Fasting to harvest results. Remember, getting healthy and losing weight takes time, dedication, and perseverance. It is not something that can be done overnight.

WITH THAT IN MIND, there can be a few side effects that can be brought on or worsened by combining these two diets:

- **Pre-Existing Health Conditions:** Both of these diets can be stressful on anyone's body. Yet, if you have diabetes, heart disease, or any circulatory issues, do not start either before consulting your doctor.

- **Withdrawal-like Symptoms:** Since one or both of these practices can be extremely taxing on your body, it makes sense that you might have some withdrawal-like symptoms. These symptoms include irritability, fatigue, headache, sour stomach, and anxiety. While this is not 'dangerous' as it is only the withdrawal from sugar, it can put a person in a dangerous situation, if they suddenly feel ill. This is why it is important to watch yourself and ease into anything you do as a senior. Remember,most seniors are not only working with how their body naturally feels, but also how the medications and other health issues react to the diets. That means there is a lot going on in your body, so allowing your body to adapt slower is a much safer bet.

DO NOT MISCONSTRUE; it is not necessary to do both the keto diet and Intermittent Fasting to reach ketosis. Seniors as well as people of all ages need to take care of themselves but they need to ensure they are not dieting themselves to death. While the keto diet and Intermittent Fasting is not dangerous, those with the following conditions or issues need to be very careful. Whether it is getting disoriented and falling, or having these side effects triggering another medical issue, overdoing your capabilities can be dangerous. Tread carefully when taking part in either or both of these diets.

ALSO, before you do anything, especially something as drastic as the keto diet, along with Intermittent Fasting, talk to your doctor. Listen to what your doctor has to say. If you are advised against one, the other, or both, do not do it!

IF YOU WANT a book on Keto I made one! Click here!

CONCLUSION

There is an endless list of different diets that people try and even more home-remedy methods of getting healthier. Some of these methods are completely unhealthy and some are contradictory to one another. Often, certain methods work on different people better than they work on others.

However, the important thing to note is that the vast majority of these different methods have one thing in common; eating less. To reiterate, it is important to maintain a healthy diet, inclusive of fruits, vegetables and plenty of water. Any diet that you want to make into a long-term commitment should include these essential elements. If not, there is still a possibility you will lose weight but there is not a possibility that you will become healthier.

Remember that.

Intermittent Fasting is effective because it only limits when you can eat. That leaves plenty of room for healthy choices, but it also helps solidify an eating schedule you can stick to.

Before starting this, or any diet, though, consult your doctor.

FAQ

Is there a good time to fast?

This is highly debated and ultimately, most Intermittent Fasting methods leave this up to the individual. Based on the research though if you have unfavorable insulin resistance, or you have issues with glucose, you might want to fast in the afternoon. The reason is that our insulin resistance gets better as the day continues.

This is more of an unconventional method but for some people, it works very well and enables them to receive the benefits of Intermittent Fasting without sacrificing their quality of life.

"Your body can't deal with nutrients (glucose) as efficiently later in the day, so you might as well give your body a break from glucose then," Dr. Krista Varady says. "Early in the day, your body is primed and ready to deal with an influx of nutrients."

For people who are using alternate-day fasting, participants have the option of having a single meal or dividing their roughly 500 calories over two or three small meals.

Do I have to eat before I work out?

There is a lot of debate over this within the health and weight loss community. However, the general consensus is that each person needs to decide for themselves. Some people feel the results of their workout routine is amplified by working out while fasting. They believe they get more energy and are able to work longer and harder. For some, you would think exercising while in a fasted state makes them superhuman.

Yet, there are others who believe that if they could not get through a workout without having something in their stomach. Therefore, there are still a large amount of healthy people in the world who do not believe it is good for your body to exercise while still fasting.

Science basically rules that it is up to the person. However, for seniors, since their performance is more health-related and less performance based, be very careful if you choose to exercise before breaking your fast. While this action has been linked to accelerated weight loss, seniors have more to worry about than simply shaving the pounds. There is medications and health-related hindrances that might make exercising before breaking their fast more consequential than the discomfort of being hungry.

Therefore, as this guide has often insisted, it is best to ask a doctor what would be best for you and what to expect before

Can I take my Medication without breaking fast?

The short answer: Yes.

While it is extremely important for seniors to keep to their specific medication schedules, this is not a practice that is specific to seniors or any age group. Modern medicine has come a long way in the past few decades and even though fasting is healthy in the long term, medications keep us alive to see the long term.

If a medication can be taken without food and must be taken in the morning (or otherwise during your fast), you should be good to go. The problem arises when you need to take medication with food, during your fasting time.

Whether this is the case or not, though, it is important to discuss this with your doctor before starting an Intermittent Fasting routine. The most important thing though, is to not miss medication because of fasting. That could cause medical emergencies that could be immediately life-threatening.

Can I put lemon in my water/tea?

Many people have a hard time drinking copious amounts of water without putting anything in it. This is definitely a hindrance for many people who would otherwise be okay with Intermittent Fasting. Fortunately, when it comes to water and even tea, diet participants are not stuck with drinking their preferred beverages without anything else to inspire the flavor.

Lemon is a popular, healthy choice for flavoring water and tea. Lucky for people who are accustomed to this, regular, unflavored lemon water is approved for consumption during fasting. This means that research has found zero effects on the fasted state.

However, the state of the lemon is important. If lemons are crushed or squeezed empty, then your lemon water is more like lemonade. Squeezing a lemon is iffy because some experts believe that any portion of the lemon (other than juice) getting in the drink could break your fast.

It is believed and accepted that 1-2 teaspoons of lemon juice in your water is not going to break a fast. Thus, getting pure lemon juice, from a bottle, or squeezed from a lemon, without any of the actual lemon skin does not affect fasting.

Actually, lemon juice is very good for your body. Among other benefits, lemon juice is great for the prolonged health of a person's kidneys and helps with cleansing of the liver.

Furthermore, when pure lemon juice is combined with apple cider vinegar, this fast-friendly concoction is able to amplify these benefits. Here are the accepted benefits of apple cider vinegar:

- Improved kidney health
- A better balance of pH balance in the person's blood
- It stabilizes blood sugar
- Appetite suppressor

Overall, this sounds like a great alternative to just drinking water or plain tea throughout the day.

Although, the taste of apple cider vinegar might take some time to get used to, just as a warning.

What Should I Eat After My Intermittent Fast?

Eating. Even when you are trying to avoid it, food is likely going to be on your mind as much as or possibly even more than before, as you try Intermittent Fasting. Whether you are actively trying not to eat, or deciding what you are going to have after your fast is over, the fact remains that you are still thinking about food. Do not be discouraged, though. This is completely normal.

The main thing a person who is Intermittent Fasting needs to remember is once the fasting is over, you need to hone in on eating a healthy diet. Unfortunately, when you do a good job fasting, you do not want to give yourself a treat, reward, or anything that will dismiss some of the progress you made. To fast appropriately, you cannot binge on unhealthy food and expect to be healthy. Instead, it is all the more important to give yourself food that is helpful to your body's development. Yes, that means fruits and vegetables.

Of course, having a meal is important, it just cannot be a meal that is larger or otherwise different than a normal meal. If you stop your fast at 4:00 in the afternoon but you do not have dinner until later, do not cave and have dinner at 4:00pm. You can have a light snack, such as a smoothie, some fruit, or vegetables, but wait to have dinner at your normal time. However, do not have a supersized dinner. Eat a normal-sized portion dinner. You do not want to overdo it and make yourself overly full. That is going to blunt the results of your fast (and it will likely make you feel horrible.)

Fortunately, the craving for unhealthy foods should subside as the fast continues. When your body is freed from the haze of processed food and heavy sugar, it will be rejuvenated and renewed. Instead of "craving" the bad stuff, it will appreciate food that is more helpful to it. When this happens, you will likely crave food that is healthy, because your body is able to tell you what it needs, without being blinded by what it wants.

Additionally, when you break your fast, you do not want to overwhelm your body. After all, when you eat anything, your body needs to switch its source of energy. That is a process in and of itself. Giving your body a large or overly rich, sudden meal to break your fast is not doing your body or yourself any favors.

Why Do I Get a Headache When Intermittent Fasting?

Getting a headache while fasting is not a certainty but it is common. After all, your body is used to getting carbs and calories whenever it demands. While you are fasting, you are denying your body what it thinks it needs to survive. However, despite the aggravation of a fasting headache, it is not dangerous and it is not permanent.

A lot of research concerning physical side effects have come from studying the Ramadan and Yom Kippur fasting rituals. This is because the religious beliefs are the most consistent and modern types of fasting, outside of Intermittent Fasting. Research has shown that women are more susceptible to headaches while fasting than men. Yet, it is not uncommon for a man to get a fasting headache. However, scientists are finding out that the reason for the headache is not caused by what one might expect.

Despite much of the religious fasting traditions banning water and food during the fasting period, the headaches are not due to hunger or dehydration. (After all, if it was due to dehydration, Intermittent Fasting participants shouldn't have a problem because they are encouraged to drink water. Yet, this is a symptom that is found throughout all forms of fasting; both religious and wellness.

It is now suspected that many headache symptoms are due to withdrawal...from carbs and sugars. Yes, a 2018 study published in Science Direct shows evidence that there is such a crutch as a food addiction and many people suffer from it. Here are a few of the other symptoms that the study found to be a part of the withdrawl, according to FARE (Food Addict Research Education):

- **Grief:** Grief is an odd thing. People who have a food addiction are usually plagued by psychological and emotional ties to food. If nothing else, food makes them happy. Eating whatever you want is freeing and when people let that freedom get the better of them, they make a lifestyle that is dedicated to food. So, it makes perfect sense that when people cut out sugar and high-processed foods, they will feel grief. Their life, as they know it, a large portion of what they looked forward to every day is being replaced by something that does not give them the same feelings or satisfaction. Any addiction is difficult to overcome. Food is no different.
- **Depression or sadness:** Food, sugar and carbs especially, helps your mood. Not only does food make a food addict happy,

it also provides a chemical pick-me-up. In this sense, food does act just like a drug. Thus, when people are suddenly unable to indulge in this emotionally and chemically satisfying ritual, they can feel lost. Plus, with the dependency gone, the person is going to feel extremely sad and even depressed.

- **Excitabile, Irritable, and Rash:** Food, like any other addictive substance replaces feelings and desires that we do not want. An addiction placates fears, anger, and anxiety. Therefore, when that substance or sustenance is no longer an option, the idea that people have to deal with their problems themselves stresses them out. In addition to feeling depressed, grieving, and angry, people now have to navigate this whole new world without the companion that has seen them through it all. That can make them excitable, quick to irritation, and rash.

- **Social withdrawal:** Food can be a universal language; the great equalizer. Everyone loves food and regardless of our relationship with it, everyone wants to eat good food. Therefore, people readily use it to connect with other people. It serves as a common ground for everyone when the person is partaking in their favorite foods. However, without that commonality, they are lost. People who were once the life of the party can no longer partake in anything that made them such. They cannot eat or drink the way they used to and the reminder of that is everywhere, as food is a large part of our society. This could make someone be a social recluse. If they do it for long enough, that might become their default and it is hard to get someone out of that. This is why it is so important for people to have a support system when they are trying to make themselves healthier. If they do not have it, they are alienated from the rest of the world. If that is the case, why bother?

- **Anxiety:** In addition to the emotional responses that go through our brain, during the fasting process, the brain is also going through physical withdrawal. A body that is going through the fasting process, especially at the beginning is getting used to an entirely new way of living. Therefore, it is going to be on high alert for a little while, as nothing is certain anymore.

The fortunate thing about getting a headache, or any

withdrawal symptoms while fasting is that it does not last for long. The worst of it is usually over within a few days and you can always take medication or deal with a headache as you would normally. Taking aspirin and drinking water is not going to break your fast. Additionally, getting a good amount of fresh air during your fast is key to dealing with these symptoms as they arise.

Why Do I Get Cold When Intermittent Fasting?

When a person fasts, the blood flow to the person's body fat is increased. This process is called adipose tissue blood flow. When a person is obese, the bloodflow is hindered significantly. This process is part of the reason, studies suggest that diabetics or pre-diabetics have impared circulation.

While a person is fasting, more blood flow is getting to the body fat. The reason this occurs is thought to be as a way to help it travel to the person's muscles, to ease the process of burning it for fuel. Due to this increased travel to your body fat, vasoconstriction occurs in the fingertips and sometimes the toes to compensate. As long as the person does not have any circulatory issues, or takes any medication that causes vasoconstriction, this is not an abnormal or dangerous occurrence.

Is it safe for Women to partake in Intermittent Fasting?

This is more a gender-related question, than a senior-related question, as it applies to women of all ages. Although, the advice that answers this question is great advice for both men and women seniors too.

This is an interesting controversy for the Intermittent Fasting community. Yes, there are studies that say fasting has a negative impact on fertility. Those studies are not inaccurate but they are not explaining the full truth. These studies have all used the alternate-day fasting method as the basis for their research. As mentioned previously, this is the most study-specific Intermittent Fasting method to date. As such, both groups, for and against all types of Intermittent Fasting use these results to illustrate their points. This doesn't always mean that it pertains to the specific type of Intermittent Fasting the article or presentation is referring to.

Specifically when it comes to safety, the alternative is that a weekly 24-hour fast is much more applicable because it is much less prolonged. Instead of fasting every other day and eating nothing for three or four days out of the week, there is only one day that is compromised by fasting. This has proven to be a lot nicer to a woman's menstrual cycle.

Additionally, women should not fast at all if they are pregnant or breastfeeding. While women should maintain a healthy diet while pregnant and breastfeeding, they are not under any circumstances advised to fast for any length of time.

Now, as it pertains to seniors, they do not have to worry about fertility, pregnancy, or breastfeeding. (Even a senior man who has a child-bearing wife is not going to affect his wife's fertility by Intermittent Fasting.) So, the conventional reasons women might be advised against fasting no longer truly apply.

The advice for women, however, is the same for seniors, with medical clearance, that are still leery about Intermittent Fasting; start slow and build your way up. You don't want to overdo it and either have a medical emergency or just develop a negative feeling toward fasting as a whole. If you work your way up, progressively fasting for longer, instead of diving right in, you will be more successful due to these factors:

- **You will be able to set and accomplish mini goals.** Setting and achieving mini-goals is great because gives you a sense of accomplishment. Instead of working extremely hard toward one big goal, you will be able to have small victories, which will make the path to your ultimate destination far more enjoyable.
- **You will be able to change your lifestyle.** Changing your lifestyle to be healthier and less dependant on food is hard. Anything you do that is different than what you are

used to will be hard to get used to. Change makes most of us uncomfortable; even if it is for our own good. To help ease the burden of a large, all-consuming change to your lifestyle, it is better to make smaller changes over a period of time. That way, you will still be working toward your ultimate goal but you will not have to endure such a shock to your system. For seniors, this can also be a smart move medically. Even though your body might respond well to the ultimate change, it might not be good to force such a large change on your body immediately.

- **The change has a better chance of lasting.** If you implement a change slowly and allow that change to morph into a lifestyle change, it is much easier to keep implementing that change. Working up to that ultimate goal offers milestones. That way, instead of resorting back to your old ways, if something is not working with a new, smaller change, you have a baseline of comfortability along your smaller changes that you can return to. Then, you can work your way back up again from there, instead of going all the way back to where you started.

Cognitive Dissonance: This is a term used in psychology to define conflicting thoughts; usually brought on when a person's belief differs from the new information that they have received. It is a form of denial that causes the person to reject the new information, even if it is correct. This relates to weight loss, as both a defense mechanism, which support unhealthy eating behaviors.

Noradrenaline: This is a chemical that is released into our body to awaken our fight or flight energy. When our body feels as though we need energy, our levels of Noradrenaline are elevated. While this is not going to make us fearful, it will give us the energy to continue on, in order to find food, when we are fasting. This is why people who are fasting report having a lot more energy, because our body is using this Noradrenaline instead of being placated with our overabundance of food.

Ketones: Ketones are water-soluble molecules that are produced by your body's liver, curated from fatty acids when your body is low on food. This happens when a person is fasting, on a carbohydrate-restricted diet, starving, or during prolonged, intense exercise. Basically, this is the chemical that burns fat and turns it into energy.

Triiodothyronine: This thyroid hormone is also known as T3 and helps the body control growth, metabolism, body temperature, and heart rate. When a person's levels of T3 is low, weight gain and constipation is common. When a person's T3 levels are high, this results in an unusually quick heartbeat, diarrhea and weight loss. To remain healthy, a person wants to have a median level of triiodothyronine in their body. This ensures that all the physiological aspects of growth and rate remain normal.

Vasoconstriction: Vasoconstriction is the narrowing or constriction of blood vessels. When the body feels this is necessary small muscles in the walls of the blood vessel press in, creating something like a dam. This causes the blood flow to slow or become completely blocked. This occurs during fasting so that more blood can be available to move the stored fat to areas of the body where it can be used for fuel.